Gold and the Phi...

Treating Chronic Physical and Mental Illness with Mineral Remedies

Dr Peter Grünewald

Mike Reiners
Oct. 28, 2003

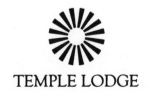

TEMPLE LODGE

Temple Lodge Publishing
Hillside House, The Square
Forest Row, East Sussex
RH18 5ES

www.templelodge.com

Published by Temple Lodge 2002

A catalogue record for this book is available from the British Library

ISBN 1 902636 31 7

Cover art by Christiane Grünewald. Cover design by S. Gulbekian
Typeset by DP Photosetting, Aylesbury, Bucks.
Printed and bound by Cromwell Press Limited, Trowbridge, Wilts.

CONTENTS

One should not slavishly follow nature. The doctor should, it is true, learn all he can from nature; but he must also be an artist, and develop nature further. Paracelsus sees true remedies not in what one takes directly from nature but in new fusions created in nature's spirit. Thus Paracelsus looks forward to an epoch in medicine in which such new products are applied as effective remedies. What is needed is nothing less than developing nature further. But the time will come when students of spiritual science will work, chemically, in harmony with evolving nature, not with what has already evolved.

Rudolf Steiner, Berlin, October 1906, GA 96

FOREWORD

This book is the result of many years' meditation, contemplation, study and research, using quantitative as well as qualitative (intuitive) methods. Although Peter Grünewald's work is based on the spiritual scientific findings of the polymath Rudolf Steiner, *Gold and the Philosopher's Stone* brings forward original and unique ideas which have been pioneered by the author. In this sense it is a development of anthroposophical medicine, not merely a commentary or condensing of previously published research. Its ideas will be of interest to doctors as well as homeopaths and other practitioners of complementary therapies, students of esoteric ideas (in particular, of course, alchemy), and to some extent patients.

As Dr Grünewald would be keen to emphasize, any research of this kind is dependent on the collaboration of colleagues. The author has worked closely with his fellow doctors in the Anthroposophical Medical Association and the Medical Section of the School of Spiritual Science for the last 14 years, and is grateful for their valuable help, ideas and feedback.

In publishing this work, we hope it will act as a catalyst for further original research and development of a spiritual medicine, which is desperately needed for humanity's further development.

Sevak Gulbekian
March 2002

ACKNOWLEDGEMENTS

The author would like to express his thanks to the friends and colleagues who gave help and assistance during the writing of this book. Special thanks go to:

Cotswold Chine School, whose generous financial support has made the publishing of this book possible.

Further: David Jones (bursar), Marguerite Wood (editor), the late John Wood, Matthew Barton (translator), Shirley Challis (pharmacist at Weleda UK), Dr Andrew Maendl (general practitioner), Dr Simon Roth (paediatrician), Dr Reinhard Schwarz (paediatrician), Dr Marga Hogenboom (general practitioner), Dr Stephan Geider (general practitioner), Dr Magdalena Isler (paediatrician), Simon Stay, Claire Kunze.

Very special thanks go to my wife Christiane and my children Katharina and Johannes for their support and endurance.

INTRODUCTION

This study examines underlying spiritual aspects of a constitutional therapy, as a rationale for the treatment of chronic physical, neurological, developmental, emotional, behavioural and mental conditions and illnesses, using medicines from the mineral kingdom.

This constitutional treatment, which can be complemented by other remedies, centres on a system of nine main minerals and one nosode:

Silica, Aurum metallicum, Phosphorus;
Ferrum sidereum, Arsenicum album, Stibium metallicum;
Calcium carbonicum, Carbo vegetabilis, Sulphur.
Tuberculinum.

I will trace these ten substances on their paths through the human organism, and demonstrate their indications, effects and interactions; a spiritual and alchemistic understanding of the working of these substances will be developed based on anthroposophical medical research.

With the help of these mineral remedies and the nosodal preparation (see below) I have been treating chronic physical, emotional, neurological, developmental, psychological and psychiatric conditions such as: affective disorders, chronic paranoid schizophrenia, behavioural problems, personality disorders, phobia, neurosis, ADD, Tourette syndrome, autism and Asperger's syndrome, as well as ME, MS, rheumatoid arthritis, eczema, allergies and recurrent infections. Their wide and universal effect as 'polychrests' means they can be used in a wide range of different illnesses and conditions, indirectly—though nevertheless effectively—treating specific illnesses by addressing the underlying psychosomatic pattern, called the 'constitution'.

This approach treats medical conditions as an imbalance of the polar tendencies to illness present in every human being, which are kept in dynamic balance within the healthy individual. Illness and crisis are here understood as a temporary or persistent lack of balance; the healing process lies in the empowerment of the 'I' of the patient to (re)create (lost) balance. The constitutional remedies developed here are designed to stimulate the re-establishment of this dynamic balance of polar psychological and physical tendencies, through the potentized compound preparation's archetypal image of this balance.

This research aims to develop a therapeutic approach and technique occupying a middle ground between the tendency in mainstream medicine to select treatment based on the nature of illness and the tendency in homoeopathy to base treatment mainly on the very personal accounts of individual patients.

Mainstream treatment tends to treat illness by countering symptoms or by substituting missing substances, while classical homoeopathic treatment treats patients' very individual mental and physical symptoms according to the principle that like is cured with like. Mainstream medical interventions as well as anthroposophical medical treatment can be successfully complemented by the remedial compositions outlined in this book.

This study is based on my therapeutic experience as a general practitioner and as a medical advisor for children and adults with learning difficulties, emotional and behavioural problems, and mental health problems.

At the end of this book you will find references and quotes, most of them from lectures by Rudolf Steiner.*

A further publication on the science and practice of the constitutional treatment of chronic physical and mental illnesses, using the system of nine mineral remedies and one nosode outlined above, is planned in the near future. This will contain a collection of audited case studies, based on instructive clinical experiences drawn from actual medical practice.

---

* The late John Wood translated the cycle of esoteric lectures (GA 265). This translation is not yet published.

Excerpts of the following lectures have been taken from his translation:

Leipzig 13.10.1906, Munich 21.5.1907 and Stuttgart 14.6.1921, as well as Hella Wiesberger's essay on the Hiram-St John individuality (GA 265).

Excerpts from the lectures of 16.12.1904 and 29.5.1907 are taken from *The Temple Legend and the Golden Legend*, Rudolf Steiner Press, London 1997, originally GA 93, also translated by John Wood.

All other quotes from Rudolf Steiner were translated by Matthew Barton.

1. THE SPIRITUALIZATION OF THE INHERITED PHYSICAL ORGANIZATION AND THE DEVELOPMENT OF THE CONSCIOUSNESS SOUL

The Origin of the Physical Body and the Forces of Heredity

The physical body is a system of forces, which give rise to the human form (*Gestalt*). According to Rudolf Steiner the physical body originates from a very early phase of human evolution, namely, Old Saturn (see *Occult Science*[1]). Beings, who had placed their warmth-substance at its disposal as will-substance, participated in the building of the physical body. In this way it was possible to form the physical germ of the body. The physical organism then passed through various stages of Earth evolution. Here I shall focus on the stage of the earth's evolution called Lemuria. This stage is referred to frequently in religious mythology, for instance in the Old Testament, as the Fall of Man. The earth was of a quite different composition at that time. The mineral kingdom was not in its present form, but airy, watery and half-solid states gradually evolved out of a condition of warmth.

An event took place during these times involving the separation of the moon from the earth. The departure of the moon allowed densification to a mineral-solid condition. The solid mineral substances that came into existence were not only present externally in the earth's natural surroundings but were also components of the human being, laid down in the skeletal system. These forces of solidification of the earth, which developed during Lemurian times, are comparable with a certain phase of embryonic development. Initially the embryo is gelatinous, and the bones gradually crystallize out from the head, via the midline, to the periphery. Calcareous substances precipitate out of the bloodstream into the mineral state.

The minerals have developed out of living organisms and not vice versa, as is the prevailing view of contemporary science. The mineral realm is formed as a dead product of the living—like a shell from a mollusc, or coal and silica forming from the skeletons of plants. This mineralization process of the earth during Lemurian times has had its effects on man. One of these is that the soul-spiritual organization of human beings relates to their bodily organization on earth in a way that allows a kind of severance from spirit or cosmic consciousness, enabling a spiritual death process to take place. Thus in human evolution a consciousness of birth and death arose involving an extinguishing of awareness of the spiritual world.

Another event in Lemurian times was the separation of the sexes, giving rise to animal and human heredity. Only when individuals of two different sexes unite can individuality arise on the one hand, i.e. daughters and sons are different from the parents, and on the other hand the passing on of certain genes comes about.

In those times, forces of heredity were not as degenerate as they are today, but were an expression of cosmic forces. People saw to it that in succeeding generations of cultural evolution the 'blood', i.e. heredity, was kept pure. Indeed, the Jewish people have a deep knowledge of the forces of heredity—for instance, the fact that the forces of heredity pass more strongly from the first to the third generation than they do from the first to the second. According to Jewish tradition descendants bear the name of their grandfather. On the other hand, they know that belonging to the Jewish people is attributable above all to the forces of inheritance of the mother. In the twelve tribes of Israel, which at the same time were hereditary lineages, cosmic archetypal powers were passed on which can be traced to the zodiac—Judah the Lion, for instance. These lineages enabled the people who were born into them to perceive their particular cultural tasks, for example priestly service. In this way spiritual tasks were to a large extent sustained by heredity.

Individualizing the 'Physically Inherited Model Body'

Rudolf Steiner described a 'physically inherited model body' (*Modelleib*). This is the physical body, originating from the stream of inheritance.[2] This is a kind of model, similar to a template on which the higher members of the human being can build up and renew the entire body. Are the forces of the individual strong enough to change parts of the model body? Or are they weak, so that by the seventh to ninth year the physical body still remains a true copy of the inherited bodily model? For the second seven years of life Rudolf Steiner referred to the 'body of the human personality'. This is a physical body which more or less exhibits the gestures, physical shape and physiognomy of the forces of the actual individuality.

Work on changing the forces of physical inheritance takes place mainly in childhood, though even as adults we have the possibility of transforming the burden of inheritance through personal development. However, we should not underestimate this burden, even for adults. Heredity plays an important part in human spiritual development. During childhood development it becomes a kind of resistance factor, enabling the individuality to grow strong through the battle between the self-determining human 'I' and the determining factors of inheritance and adaptation to environmental influences.

The process of individualization of the physical body begins when the individuality, encompassed by its supersensible sheaths, connects with the embryo. Rudolf Steiner describes the physical body of the embryo—which is strongly influenced by inheritance, and which the child inhabits until the age of seven—as the 'model' that is then reworked through the activity of astral body and ego. This body formed through the forces of heredity acts only as a model for the building up of a new physical vessel, which may then be termed the 'human personality body'.[3] In this reworking and transformation of the physical body, the forces of heredity of the 'model body' are overcome or rather metamorphosed, so that from the time of the change of teeth heredity is no longer really an active force. However, depending on the power to transform the body that an individual brings from pre-birth existence, the ego and the astral body will be either more or less faithful to the model in building a new physical embodiment. In strong individualities, therefore, there is only a slight resemblance between the 'model body' and the 'human personality body'.[4] (This transformation can for example be observed in the change of facial features, as well as in increasing individualization of movement and gesture, further expressing the child's individuality.)

The degree of strength of individualization is dependent on knowledge and deeds gained in one's previous life, as well as between death and a new birth. In after-death existence the sense-world experiences of a previous life transform into knowledge and capacity for building and transforming a new body in the next incarnation. Paucity of sense experiences lead in a subsequent life, through lack of knowledge of the laws for building up a new physical organization, to pathological formations of individual organs of the model body.[5]

The ego's experience in the Saturn sphere between death and a new birth is of decisive importance for its power of individualization. Here, in union with the beings of the First Hierarchy, and together with all the human souls karmically connected to it, this human ego structures the macrocosmic archetypal image of its physical embodiment. The so-called spirit seed arises here as head organization transformed from the metabolic limb system of the previous life.

The spherical structure of this head organization, however, is initially spread right out into the whole cosmos. The spirit seed contains form-structuring powers for the next incarnation, and is the head organization's spiritual predisposition. As such it bears the formative forces with which the child later builds up its body. On the other hand it is also woven from purely moral substance. In descending through the planetary spheres, it increasingly draws itself in and together, and receives from the beings of the Second and Third Hierarchies the spiritual form of the rhythmic and metabolic-limb systems.[6] At the moment of conception, when the human ego dwells with its astral body in the moon sphere so as to form its etheric body from the cosmic ether, the spirit seed releases itself from the ego and unites with the embryo.[7] Around the seventeenth day after conception, the ego and its sheaths then reunite with the spirit seed and participate in the embryo's development.[8] The spirit seed gradually transforms into the actual human form and is then termed the 'phantom body'.

Now, as suggested above, the power of the ego for individualizing the inherited physical body depends on the individuality's passage through the world beyond Saturn. Conscious activity in building up the spirit seed changes into the capacity for transforming this inherited body during the first seven years of life. If the human ego has the strength to remain highly conscious during the process of developing the spirit seed in union with other spiritual beings—which depends on capacities gained in the previous incarnation—it will then enter the next incarnation as a strong individuality. (The expressions 'strong' or 'weak' individuality has nothing to do with the intellectual brilliance, talents or possibly advanced spiritual development that an individual has attained in the course of his life. In this context it refers only to the degree of ability to individualize the physical body, while gifts and talents come to expression in an individual's spirit self-hood.) The ego is then able to diverge a good deal from the inherited model in building up its second physical body, the 'human personality body'. This capacity manifests in a comparatively early retrieval during the embryonic period of the spirit seed that has been sent on ahead, which means that the ego participates from a relatively early point in building up the body, perhaps even before the seventeenth day after conception.[9]

It can happen that a human ego has only gained weak powers of individualization in the Saturn and zodiacal spheres. When it then unites through incarnation with the inherited model body, it can build up from it a new physical body—but, in so doing, it must adhere closely to the model. The second physical body will then be very similar to the first. (This can also happen if the individuality decides to build a second physical body that is even more similar to the parent-body than the first one.)[10]

What is then formed does not derive from the physical forces of heredity themselves, since these are no longer active after the change of teeth.[11] But during the first seven years the forces of heredity work strongly and formatively upon the weak individuality, so that it is compelled to form the second body as these forces dictate, possibly also including the formation of pathological organ structures. When the higher members are freed from the task of forming this second body (at the change of teeth) and become available for soul activity, defects in the body's structure also cause disturbances in soul-spiritual development, for instance in the form of so-called will-defects.[12]

(We can, for example, discern this 'continued influence of inherited disposition' in children who have not, or only insufficiently, undergone childhood illnesses. The processes described here really require a new understanding of so-called inherited illnesses and genetic syndromes. The 'expressivity' of inherited disposition is then seen to be a question of the ego's power of individualization, i.e., how closely the ego must adhere to its model when building up the new body.)

The Effects of Genetic Forces (Heredity) and of Adaptation

In considering the four members of man's being—physical body, etheric body, astral body (the bearer of the soul forces), and ego—the following distinctions can be discerned.[13]

Firstly, forces emerge from the physical body that bind life and soul processes to the physical. These are above all genetic forces. In cases of genetic disorders, for example, the ego organization is too loosely integrated and unable to attach itself sufficiently to the other members of the individual's being. This means that to some extent the 'I' is no longer able to take hold of the other members. This is a similar situation to the relationships between the different bodily sheaths or members which prevail in the animal kingdom, where the force of the 'I' has to work from outside as the animals' group souls. In people with strongly inherited characteristics or with genetic disorders, astral and etheric bodies are too deeply embodied within their physical organization. This can manifest itself in material forces determining consciousness and life processes too strongly. This configuration can be observed too in genetically determined physical diseases, like hypertension, diabetes and others, as well as in genetic syndromes as different as Down's syndrome, Williams syndrome, Martin Bell syndrome and others.

At the level of mind and consciousness, people with a predominance of the constitution outlined above can often feel themselves to be victims of their own physically determined instincts, drives, and desires. In extreme cases, they might easily feel cut off from all spiritual experience.

Secondly, a person's ego organization can be too strongly connected to soul and life processes; and all three are to some extent disconnected from the physical body, which as a consequence remains untransformed. A person with predominance of this constitution will often feel disconnected from the physical world, but can be very open to one-sided spiritual experiences. This person might cut him/herself off from anything material, turn away from the world of the senses, and reduce their food intake through fasting in order to close off the bridge between their physical body and the outside world. Other people might mimic, copy or mirror the environment in their behaviour, without truly individualizing it (adaptation). They often feel overwhelmed and too strongly determined by their social environment.

It is the express task of the human being to create a balance between the spiritual and the physical. Only in this way can mankind further its spiritual evolution. Mankind's spiritual evolution proceeds through the individual transforming inherited forces and environmental influences; true imitation is the first step in this process during the first seven years of a child's life.

The Struggle Between Individuality and Genetic Forces

The concept of 'penetrance' or 'expressivity' describes the battle of the individuality against genetic forces. In using these terms people acknowledge that certain genetic information (like the trisomy 21 in Down's syndrome) can express itself strongly in some cases or only very slightly in others. The expression of certain symptoms of the syndrome varies considerably in different individuals with the same genetic condition. This distinction between phenotype and genotype raises the question of the extent or intensity to which the genes bring about external appearance and their internal effects (consciousness). It is this intensity, dependent on the forces of individualization, which is referred to as penetrance or expressivity. So when certain pathological genetic forces are present and encounter very strong forces of individualization, the 'I' (self) is in a position to extensively transform the forces of inheritance. In such a case, what is present in the genes expresses itself only very weakly. And in the opposite situation the genes express themselves much more strongly.

Transforming Heredity and Adaptation Through Imitation

In childhood development, we find many examples of inherited behaviour patterns, like primitive reflexes and spontaneous movements of the limbs, or activities and behaviour based on metabolic functions (such as hunger, thirst etc.). In the course of time some of these inherited behaviour patterns are transformed or disappear as the result of coordinated movements acquired through imitation.

Through imitation children learn to internalize certain movement patterns in their environment in such a way that they become able to act according to these patterns. The inherited motor reflexes are overcome to the extent that these movement patterns are assimilated, internalized and repeated imitatively.

This brings about the development of the brain and cerebral structures. But the child does not stop there. As well as imitating gestures and human activities, thereby overcoming inherited movement patterns, a new faculty unfolds—through imitation of movement patterns and behaviour, the child develops the ability for self-expression.

Thus imitative movement becomes transformed into 'individualized movement'—for instance, facial expression—and expresses what the child has developed out of his inner being.

As a result of the process of internalization and individualization that results from imitation, activities can unfold whose developmental laws are not embedded in the genes, such as walking, talking and thinking. This needs to be emphasized, because nobody would be able to walk, speak and think if they did not have other people around them. In human beings these faculties are only acquired through social contact with others.

The moral quality of actions by people in the child's immediate environment is of special importance here. This moral substance of people surrounding the child has a nurturing or deforming effect on the way the body develops. Still, the child's ego selects during sleep those impressions that have an up-building effect. However, the capacity to select impressions also, in turn, depends on the power of individualization that the ego has attained in its existence between death and a new birth. Moral impressions of the child's environment carried through sleep do not only affect the body's development, but also, via the body, exert an influence on the formation of habits and the life of soul.

Thus forces of heredity encounter formative forces exerted by the moral quality of the child's environment. Heredity and adaptation have a formative and determining effect on the body's development during the first seven years. Into this influence of polar forces the child's ego intervenes, in its striving for freedom, to individualize the body's substance and forces and the environment's moral substance in harmony with the capacities the individuality has brought with it. Defects arise in the formation of the second body if the power of individualization is weak, and/ or if the inherited substance is pathological, and/or the child's environment has no moral quality. When the higher members become partially freed, these defects also lead to disturbances in the human being's soul and social development at later stages of life.

Imitation involves a twofold process. On the one hand behaviour patterns are internalized and on the other hand contact with the environment, with the mother and father, is developed in such a way that behaviour is not only copied but becomes so united with the soul-spiritual essence of the other person that the morality which expresses itself in this speaking and doing is absorbed and internalized. In uniting with the soul-spiritual nature of another person, the child's soul is engaged in a morally formative process. Through imitation the child gradually represses its own forces of heredity and transforms them, but also individualizes behavioural patterns internalized from the environment.

Rudolf Steiner indicated that the possibility of individualization arises especially in the first seven years, during which the forces of heredity can to some extent be changed and overcome. These forces offer resistance to those of individualization. A kind of battle goes on. When the soul-spiritual element unites with the embryo during its development and comes up against the forces of inheritance, which are foreign to its nature, an intense struggle takes place between the forces of the individual and those of heredity. The strength of the forces of the individual determines whether the child will be able to change its physical appearance, its gestures and its physiognomy around the seventh, eighth or ninth year in such a way that they become increasingly unlike the corresponding characteristics inherited from its parents in stature, constitution, physiognomy, gestures and facial expression. (This transformation is usually more or less incomplete, however, and a residue of untransformed inherited influences is always left.)

Pathology of the Imitation Process

We must also discriminate between imitation and conditioning or mere reflection. In curative education we come across a certain group of children, so-called autistics, who have a tendency to copy the movements of others exactly. It is a kind of process of reflection. There is no individualization, no real internalization. They are incredibly good mimics of birdcalls, for instance. Their condition demonstrates a disturbance in imitative behaviour, which leads to an incomplete transformation of inheritance with consequences for the spiritual development of the child—an inability to develop the consciousness soul later in life.

A poorly individualized model body has repercussions for spirit-soul development in the biographical stage of the consciousness soul, during the sixth seven-year period.[14]

The consciousness soul, developing through the work of the ego organization on the physical body, is one of the three soul members (together with the sentient and the mind soul), and, at the same time, the provisional product of transformation arising through the work of the ego on the physical spirit body, on the evolutionary path towards Spirit Man (*Atma*).[15] Its development is substantially prepared through the individualizing and reworking of the model body and the moral substance of the social environment. If both these forces (inheritance and environment) overpower a child's ego, the individual will later find it hard, in developing the consciousness soul, to liberate the will in two directions from the physical organization. In this case two pathological forms of moral development arise: on the one hand a fixed and inflexible moral system that has adopted its beliefs from the environment without really working them through; and on the other hand, a moral blindness that makes it impossible for the individual to properly integrate himself and his own will impulses into the moral context of the world. The tendency to these pathologies is already perceptible in childhood. They naturally appear in all degrees of severity and also in various combinations. (One may think here, for instance, of autism and obsessive syndromes on the one hand, and kleptomania and psychopathic illness on the other.) Such tendencies to disturbed development can be balanced out in later life through education, therapy and the path of esoteric training.[16]

The Transformation of Inheritance and Adaptation Through Intuition

In further development during childhood imitation loses its importance and strength in the process of transforming inheritance. New skills and activities have to be acquired, which are like a metamorphosis of the early childhood activity of imitation.

Rudolf Steiner describes three future developmental stages of consciousness—Imagination, Inspiration and Intuition—which have started to be experienced in our time, usually as forces which fill our daily life of thinking, feeling and willing with truthfulness and spirit presence. Through meditative activity they can be enhanced and brought to increased awareness.

These states of consciousness are the result of the connection of human consciousness with different regions of the spiritual world. In the early stages of mankind's development they were originally the expression of man's atavistic relationship to the spiritual world and its beings. In order to gain the potential of freedom and independence, man had to lose this faculty, thus developing an earthbound consciousness, which can base its motives of action on scientific knowledge, common sense, self-determination and love. Developing the faculties of Imagination, Inspiration and Intuition is therefore not falling back into atavistic states of consciousness (as one might try to do with the help of drugs or inappropriate meditation techniques), but rather the result of a disciplined inner training path, which extends modern scientific consciousness into the realm of perceiving the world of spiritual beings and forces. In this process of perception of the spirit, clarity of thinking, judgement, healthy common sense, independence and control must not be lost. Human consciousness can thus become, in all independence and freedom, a bridge between spiritual and physical worlds. (See: *How To Know Higher Worlds; Occult Science; Philosophy of Freedom.*)

Intuition is a stage of the evolution of human consciousness, which will arise, *inter alia*, through the coming into existence of a capacity for morally creative thinking and love. Intuition will gradually develop and is in progress at the present time. It can be developed in two directions.

Firstly it is developed through morally creative thinking, when will activity is evolved in a sense-free thinking process, which gives thinking a new direction not influenced by sense perception or past experiences. This creates social future in the form of moral intuitions within one's thinking and is the first of four steps of developing freedom. (See: *Philosophy of Freedom*.) By developing sense-free thinking, as is possible for example through a systematic practice and study of anthroposophy, the will is partially emancipated from its organic root in the body, and becomes active instead in the formation of thoughts and ideas. This will-imbued, sense-free thinking is a source of freely derived moral intuitions. It loosens the inflexibility of moral concepts by permeating the light-related pole of reason with the warmth of inner will activity.

Secondly, Intuition arises through activity that enables a person to rest lovingly in the being of another person, so that the being of the other person speaks from within him. Modern psychology calls this empathy, the first echoes of Intuition. One becomes united with other beings and their inner life. In returning to oneself, one gains an inward experience, created as 'after images' (Imagination) in the feeling and will life, of reactions arising from this uniting with another being. A loving devotion to the phenomena of the sense-world or towards another person can enable the light-filled element of thinking to stream down into the dark, but warm, will region, and illuminate it. In this process the will itself is cultivated in a way that enables it to lift itself out of the sphere of organic need and bodily influence, and, penetrated by thought, unite harmoniously with the moral context and meaning of the world.[17]

Pure sense-free thinking, as Rudolf Steiner described in his *Philosophy of Freedom*, as well as loving devotion to the other person (unity of beings in empathy) are the two most important sources of Intuition in our time. These two activities are at the same time the basis of the development of the consciousness soul.

The first path of practice gives rise to an experience of freedom in will-imbued thinking, through the creative process of moral intuitions. In the second path, moral intuitions find their way into the world via their connection with the lower, outward-focused will organization, becoming effective motives for action.

The connecting link of this dual metamorphosis of thinking and willing can be found in the sphere of the rhythmic system. This is where moral love and moral intuitions—which still have the character of ideas—develop and transform into living ideals. On the other hand we open ourselves through our rhythmic system to the moral content of natural phenomena that can be experienced in the sense world.

The Forces of Intuition

The forces of Intuition strengthen the human I so that it can transform and enliven the human physical body through the etheric body.[18] The effect of the 'I' on the lower members of man takes place in imitation in childhood in the same way as later on in life in developing the consciousness soul or in the process of developing Intuition through sense-free thinking or love.

Intuition and consciousness–soul development allow a spiritualization of the physical body.

The child partially completes this spiritualization process of the physical body in its first seven years of life. Many faculties we develop as children are in a certain sense lost when we become adults. Our power of judgement develops, our experiences become more selective. We begin to assign more importance to our own soul life than to our environment. Even so, the transformation occurring in the first seven years is preparation for the development of higher faculties such as free moral creativity in the consciousness–soul epoch.

This is exemplified by the case of an autistic adult who could copy movements very well and could also speak but who was unable to develop independent morality. He always asked others how he should behave. He saw his morality only as a reflection of his surroundings.

Transformation of the forces of heredity during the first seven years enables the individual in physical embodiment to attain a personal morality, which can be realized in love for another person.

The Results of Overcoming the Forces of Heredity and Adaptation

As human beings we must strive to transform and individualize the forces of heredity and adaptation. Therein lies the possibility of unfolding from within us capacities such as love, Intuition, and independent morality. Rudolf Steiner spoke of the evolution of the consciousness soul as the product of the transformation of the physical body through the 'I'.

Does the physical body, with its forces of inertia, remain sufficiently open to the possibility of the individuality continuing to work within it in further spiritual development? Or does it become so hardened and densified through material forces (as for example treatment with drugs, fluorides, GM food, and other life-style influences) that the individuality is no longer able to work into the physical body, the body of the Word, of the senses, of morality?

Transforming Heredity and Adaptation

Anthroposophical medicine attempts to strengthen the spirit being of a patient gradually, so that it becomes able to transform the forces of heredity and adaptation. This still appears necessary after the seventh year of life, after which genetic and inherited forces continue to partly determine the functions of man's higher members in physiology and consciousness.

In anthroposophical medicine, therapy with potentized minerals can strengthen the 'I'; by encountering the spiritual aspect of a mineral medicine, the 'I' can be empowered to work in a transformative way right into the forces of heredity. The result of this therapeutic process is an enhancement of the development of the consciousness soul.

The above outlined twofold path, centred in the rhythmic organization, is the basis for a healthy development towards freedom and love at the consciousness-soul level, in equilibrium between light and warmth. It represents the beginning of the ego's conscious work of spiritualizing and enlivening the physical organization of the body, which, as phantom body, has a form or light aspect, and a strength or warmth aspect. In developing a mineral-therapy system we will examine more closely this dual aspect of the spiritual-physical organization and its equilibrium.

2. THE BREATHING PROCESS AND THE MINERAL KINGDOM AS A BASIS FOR THE DEVELOPMENT OF EGO AND PHYSICAL BODY

In our present evolutionary period, respiration is the basis of ego development in a physical body. The rhythm of this respiration has a close relation to the Platonic Year. Thus the average number of breaths an adult takes each day is 25,920 (18 breaths per minute), in other words, as many breaths in a day as there are sun years in a Platonic Year. (The Platonic Year is the period during which the spring equinox travels once through the zodiac. This so-called precession of the equinox takes place in contrary motion to the sun's passage through the zodiac in the course of a solar year. The Platonic Year lasts roughly 25,920 years.)

If, in considering the larger breathing rhythm of birth and death, we assume a 'patriarchal' life expectancy of 72 years, a human life on earth lasts one day in the Platonic Year.

And in the intermediate breathing rhythm of sleeping and waking, we pass through 25,920 sleeping/waking cycles in the course of this average lifetime of 72 years.

The numerical relation of these three rhythms to the Platonic Year is an expression of the inner connection between the microcosm man—and the ensouled and spirit-permeated life of the macrocosm. The macrocosmic rhythm is internalized in human respiration, and in the cycles of human life.

Thus respiration integrates us into the cosmos, while the rhythm of blood circulation, which tends towards metabolism, is in danger of wholly estranging us from the cosmos. After respiration has fully developed (around the twelfth year), a task of this breathing rhythm is to restrain the rhythm of circulation that is so influenced by the metabolic organization, so that the ego can create a balance in our mediating, rhythmic sphere between the cosmic forces of the head and the earthly forces of metabolism.[19] If this rhythmic equilibrium does not become established, pathology in either direction can come about. A pulse/breath ratio of 1:4 is an expression of harmonious balance, achieved by the rhythmic system between the two polar forces.

The human ego, as it strives for freedom through equilibrium, is decisively involved in sustaining this rhythmic relationship, which for man represents an archetypal healing impulse. Through this rhythmic correlation it creates the physiological basis for self-healing and development towards freedom.

In building up the human being's bodily sheaths in pre-birth existence, macrocosmic rhythms become internalized in such a way that they then unfold as microcosmic rhythms between birth and death. Yet the rhythms at work in the human organism have emancipated themselves from cosmic rhythms, and undergo a time-shift, which makes them distinct from the rhythms of the sun, moon and planets. This time-shift and susceptibility to disturbance of internalized human rhythms is a pre-requisite for becoming autonomous in respect of the Hierarchies and for developing human freedom.[20] At the same time this also allows illness and error to take root. The emotions and passions of the astral body, and the etheric body's one-sided dispositions of temperament and pathological propensities of habit, intervene in these autonomous rhythmic conditions and cause rhythmic disturbances, which can lead to illness.

The human ego owes its capacity for autonomy from natural phenomena and cosmic rhythms to the internalized force of Saturn.[21] The incarnating Saturn process emancipates us from natural forces and leads us to self-awareness. The 'heat-dispersing' and thus cooling mineralization tendencies of the incarnating Saturn process (a negative warmth process, not just the absence of warmth) implant bone formation (calcification) in man. This skeletal system, as death process in the human being, provides the basis for the ego's conscious activity.[22] The incarnating Saturn force allows time-rhythm and spatial conditions (skeletal system) to be internalized, thus enabling us to have conscious experience of time and space from within and to recognize these qualities of time and space within the outer world. At the same time, though, by being separated and cut off from the cosmos, the disposition to illness and death is implanted in us as we awaken to awareness of self and world.

Countering this incarnating (and solidifying) Saturn process is a second, excarnating (and spiritualizing) Saturn process that unfolds through warmth. This is the bearer of forces of resurrection and renewal and has a substance- and form-dissolving effect. In physiological terms this corresponds (alongside other planetary processes that are also involved) to blood formation in the bone marrow, but above all to the warmth at work in the blood process. If the excarnating Saturn process were not balanced by incarnating Saturn processes, this would lead to an inability to relate to earthly laws and social conditions and would dissolve a patient's perception of his earthly personality.

The human ego lives between the polar effect of these two Saturn processes, which are most purely expressed in activities of blood-heat and bone formation.[23] In the dual process of condensing and dispersal of warmth, the ego, which has to be the actual regulator of warmth, has a polar influence on the sheaths of man's being. The warmth process of the blood at the same time becomes the basis for that part of the ego organization which is active from the periphery to the centre in the lower organization (metabolic–limb system), the so-called peripheral ego organization that provides the impulse for purposeful activities of will. The other, cooling stream is the basis for the 'central ego', the part of the ego organization which, seated in the head (nerve–sense system), works from the centre to the periphery. This 'central ego', depending on the cold process related to light, is what provides the impulse for objective consciousness through sense perception and thought formation.[24] The harmonious balancing of upper and lower cold/warmth processes in the heart (between breathing and circulation) places these two processes in harmonious relationship to conditions of warmth in the outer world, and this enables us to locate within the heart our awareness of self and world as reflected in the physical body. The relationship of the ego's threefold existence—as central ego in the nerve–sense organization, as peripheral ego in the metabolic–limb organization and as balance-creating ego within the rhythmical system (respiration and circulation)—finds its reflection in the mineral realm. This threefold ego activity is manifest in the three main classes of mineral-substance processes, which Rudolf Steiner described along alchemical lines as Salt (nerve–sense system; solidifying, forming, cooling); Mercury (rhythmical system; breathing and circulation, harmony and balance) and Sulphur processes (metabolic–limb system; form-dissolving, warming).

On the level of consciousness Salt processes are the carriers of cognition (thinking and perceiving), Mercury processes of feeling and emotion and Sulphur processes of will-power within the human being. Salt processes have a conservational effect, relating us to the past, Sulphur processes relate us to our future potential, and only within the Mercury process do we fulfil our present life task by uniting past and future.

In order to avoid having a harmful effect on health, each mineral substance must, through ego activity, be transformed within the organism from the solid element to the level of warmth. This process of transformation underlying all mineral nourishment once more opens up mineral substance that has been transmuted into warmth to the activity and influence of spirit-beings of the First Hierarchy (which worked in the warmth substance of 'Old Saturn'). The Thrones, who are bearers of cosmic ego forces, can then work into their own most native element, that of warmth.[25] We must regard this 'mineral ego', formed from the substance of vital forces streaming in from the zodiacal world, as dwelling in the Saturn planetary sphere. This Saturn sphere is also the home of the human ego and of the communal ego of all human physical bodies.[26] It is in this sphere too that the spirit seed of the physical body of our next incarnations is formed from the transformation of our metabolic-limb systems into the spiritual-physical predispositions of our future head organization.[27]

Thus, when mineral substance is transformed into warmth through the process of digestion, or rather through the process of potentization (creating homoeopathic remedies from mineral substances) so intimately related to digestion, this substance becomes the bearer of the mineral ego's influence proceeding from the substance of the Thrones. As a result of potentizing or digesting a mineral, the evolutionary process of the mineral, condensed by stages from warmth into solid substance (a death process connected with the incarnating Saturn influence), is reversed and led on towards future evolution. In this process, mineral substance is redeemed by being conducted back (now via the second Saturn process) into the spirit entity of the substance of the Thrones. This is a process which prefigures the future evolution of the whole mineral realm; for by the end of the mineral round of our Earth evolution the activity of the human ego will have wholly transformed and individualized the mineral kingdom.[28]

Once man redeems the mineral realm through his ego, by means of art, science and social structures that reflect knowledge of the laws of the world of spirit, the redeemed mineral realm will, with the help of the Christ impulse, be resurrected in man's soul and become imperishable and enduring.[29] This will enable the human physical body to be raised up one level into the plant realm. Then the human ego will, via a physical body that has become plantlike, work in the same way at mastering and redeeming the plant realm as it has now begun to work upon the mineral realm.[30] The fruit of this redemption for the evolution of human consciousness will be an enhancement of the soul's power of love to such a degree that it becomes an encompassing power of knowledge. This is the level of Intuition that enables us to unite with beings of the world of spirit in the act of knowledge. Through Intuition man also learns to subject wholly to the power of his ego the processes of a physical organization that has become plantlike.[31] It leads him to overcome the death-consciousness that formed in Lemurian times. (This death-consciousness formed alongside respiration and the incorporation of dead mineral substance into his skeletal system.) The parallel evolving processes of, on the one hand, the formation of the mineral realm within man (skeleton) and the minerals in the outer world, and of the appearance of respiration on the other hand, were fundamental prerequisites for human incarnation into the bodily sheaths prepared by the Hierarchies.[32] It was thus that the human ego could incarnate out of the womb of the Elohim into physical manifestation. In so doing it relied both on the breathing process, and on the differentiated warmth processes of the mineral realm.

Reincarnation and karma began with ego-incarnation into a mineral-permeated physical body produced through sexual union. This development took place during late Lemurian times and throughout the Atlantean period. Consciousness of death, the expression of our sundering from a group-soul connection with the world of spirit, became the basis of our individual consciousness, of our self-awareness.

The fact that the breathing process (respiration) is the basis of ego-incarnation can also be seen from the derivation of the German word for breath—*Atem*. This comes from the word *Atma*, which means the shared, common ego of all human beings.[33]

This communal ego gradually and increasingly became individualized through incarnations and experiences within human physical bodies, so that each ego, originally part of the overall ego of humanity, developed its own individual destiny. The fruits of all its different earth experiences have been worked into the sheath nature of the astral body through the activity of the ego, and resurrected as the ego's eternal and individualized properties (Spirit Self).

Although the human ego became more and more individual from incarnation to incarnation, it could no longer sustain its self-awareness, its consciousness of identity, after death—for man's self-awareness depends upon the ego gaining a reflection of itself from a spiritual-physical body. The spiritual-physical body or phantom of man, however, had become so defective after the Fall that it nearly completely dissolved following death. When Christ, as representative of all humanity, overcame the power of death at the Mystery of Golgotha, humanity received the phantom body back again as resurrected body. Thus Christ's deed on Golgotha gave us two gifts: first the possibility of sustaining ego-consciousness even after death; and secondly, by taking up the Christ impulse into our ego, of creating a power of attraction to Christ's physical body of resurrection, which has multiplied since the Mystery of Golgotha.[34]

By the end of the mineral round of Earth evolution, when the mineral realm has been redeemed through the activity of the ego, the human being will have attained and incorporated this physical-spiritual body of resurrection. This is the plantlike physical body of which we spoke above.

At the consciousness level of Intuition attained with this development, death also loses its power over human beings. We will then live within two worlds, the physical and spiritual, with equal clarity of awareness of self and world. Once this happens death will only be a metamorphosis, and laying down our earthly body will be experienced as nothing more than an outer process.[35]

The Saturn–Sun Mystery described here, the awakening of the phantom body made possible for humanity through Christ's sacrifice on Golgotha, was prefigured through the path of initiation and the practices of Christian mystery schools. This stage of human evolution corresponds with the fourth level of the Rosicrucian school's path of initiation, termed 'Preparing the Philosopher's Stone', or 'Rhythmic Enlivening of Breath and Life'.[36] These two designations for this stage of consciousness and practice give us an inkling of the connection between the mineral world (stone) and the breathing process, which as we have seen evolved alongside one another as the basis for ego–incarnation in a physical body. In truth this stage of the path of schooling is a mystic one that works right into the physiology of the body, and also an alchemical one, that is, involving activity directed at transforming the mineral realm. The evolution of the mineral realm will also continue to run parallel with that of the human respiration process. Inasmuch as the ego actively participates in the transformation of both processes, it will awaken its own phantom body as the Christ-given body of resurrection.

But in following a Christian mystery path man should no longer directly influence the breathing process. Just as a mineral remedy or an artistic therapy only offers the ego a means of exerting a healing effect upon the physical organization through the breathing, so meditative practice for developing Intuition can only be a means whereby the ego takes hold of the breathing process. Every direct, physically orientated breathing exercise can have a harmful effect on people with Western constitutions. Practising intuitive consciousness imbued with the element of warmth and light—meditation in other words—leads, at a certain stage, to a condition in which the thoughts, feelings and will impulses experienced within the ego can work back upon the breathing process.

A breathing process taken hold of and altered by this means gives the ego the strength, mediated by the astral and etheric bodies, to work right into the physical body.[37] The physical spirit-body is thus directly transformed and enlivened.

On the other hand these exercises also gradually lead to all the same consequences for the physical body as occur very suddenly in non-initiates at the moment of death. In other words, the initiate is prefiguring death while still alive.[38] For this reason the exercises leading to Intuition can only be undertaken without harm to the initiate when they are practised with the utmost caution, and after sufficient preparation and purification of the life of the soul. The initiate thereby accomplishes an Imitatio Christi at the level of the crucifixion of Golgotha.

The connection between the mineral realm and the breathing process as it relates to the development of the ego and the physical body is of enormous significance to the doctor. On the one hand it provides important stimulus for medical research and the therapeutic impulses deriving from it; and on the other hand it allows a bridge to be built between therapeutic knowledge and the Mystery of Golgotha. It is the aim of this study to try to elaborate on this connection, to which Rudolf Steiner refers in the pastoral medicine course as a culmination of the doctor's path.[39] Later in this study we will examine therapeutic aspects specific to certain minerals, as part of a mineral system that will be developed with reference to the occult physiology of the breathing process. The basis for this will be the inner connection between human respiration and the effect of mineral substances—the alchemy of carbon that will also be subsequently described.

In summarizing the therapeutically orientated approach described in these pages, I would like to mention that the remedies raised to Saturn-warmth level through the potentization process can, by their 'cosmic-ego nature', unfold their therapeutic potential in two distinct directions: they work on the patient's ego and on his physical body.[40] They replace insufficient ego activity in particular physical organs of the body with their own ego activity.

The patient's weak ego is unburdened and freed from a pathological situation within an organ, and strengthened through confrontation with the mineral's ego nature. Through this healing process we can gain insight into the universality of remedies from the mineral kingdom. For instance, if an illness leads to a disturbance in the relationship between the ego organization and one of the other bodies, then a mineral remedy is the only therapeutic means of dealing with this disturbance.[41] The mineral transformed into warmth stimulates the ego organization, via the breathing process, to exert a healing effect on the body's disturbed relationship. If there is pathology of ego activity in the nerve-sense system, the use of 'salt-type' minerals is usually indicated. With ego activity disturbances in the metabolic-limb system, 'sulphuric minerals' will more commonly be used. The metals as 'mercury' substances have a direct effect through the rhythmic system and from there can, depending on the level of dilution, also have a healing effect on nerve-sense and metabolic-limb system activity. However, most metals only work down as far as the etheric body—apart from gold, which can extend its ego-directed effect via the etheric body right into the physical body.[42]

Nevertheless it lies in the nature of the mutual resonance between upper, central ego and lower, peripheral ego, mediated through the breathing process,[43] that the life of will can also be stimulated through a head-orientated treatment using 'salt-type' remedies, such as Conchae in high potency. The life of thinking can also be stimulated by treating the will organization with a sulphuric substance, as has been shown in curative education medical practice. But these mutual resonances demand much of the patient's ego, and therefore are all the more therapeutically fruitful. They are an expression of the dual metamorphosis and permeation of the life of thinking and of will described above (see page 13), and in spiritual terms represent a kind of archetypal healing process,[44] whose pathological counter-image can be seen in the two main tendencies of illness, either to sclerosis or inflammation.

3. THE FOURFOLD BREATHING PROCESS REFLECTED IN THE SUBSTANCE PROCESSES

In the seventh and eighth lectures of his pastoral medicine course,[45] Rudolf Steiner develops an occult physiology of the breathing process. From this I have taken what seems relevant to the theme examined here.

He starts with the breathing process that consists of inbreathing and out-breathing of gaseous substance via the lungs. 'The inhalation of O_2 and N_2 is an activity of the astral body.' The O_2 bears formative cosmic forces for the human organism. Through this inhalation process the astral body and ego can connect more strongly with the physical body during inhalation.

The 'process of exhalation' leads to the breathing out of carbon dioxide (CO_2). The exhalation process is underpinned by an 'activity of the etheric body'. The etheric body, which permeates water substance within the physical organization, repulses the astral body that connected with it during inhalation, thus loosening their connection. In other words, the astral body and ego are breathed out along with the carbon dioxide, and this is an effect of the etheric body penetrating the water organism. Some of the carbon dioxide that is not exhaled mediates the 'formative forces for digestive organs'.

Inhalation	Exhalation
O_2, N_2	CO_2
Activity of the astral body	Activity of the etheric body
Air	Water

(During sleep, when the astral body and ego have been wholly breathed out [into the cosmos], the macrocosmic astral body of the earth takes over this activity of the inhalation process within us.)

Above the centre of the air inhalation process (lung region), in the area which is primarily centred in the head, lies a 'refined breathing' which, although focused in the head, penetrates the whole human organism. The nerve-sense system carries a refined breathing that unfolds in the element of warmth and is linked with the activity of the ego. This can be termed as 'sense breathing', in which inhalation occurs through the sense organs from without, but exhalation proceeds inwards and connects with gaseous inhalation. Warmth is breathed in by the sense organs and breathed out into the interior human organization, thus linking with the process of air inhalation. This 'warmth-breathing process' in our inner organization underlies all the senses that perceive the outer world. 'Macrocosmic warmth', exhaled inwards through the senses, is at the same time also the bearer of the macrocosmic 'light, chemical and life ether', which are only allowed certain degrees of entry into the organism, while the warmth ether permeates the whole organism.

Below the gaseous respiration lies a breathing process, which, in contrast to the latter, watery process, represents a 'coarsening'. This is the digestive process, which can also be termed a 'metabolic breathing'. This is connected to the 'activity of the physical body', and occurs in the solid, earth element.

Each of these physiological processes is connected with certain distinct planetary forces, which in their representation within the human organism regulate certain soul-life qualities, life processes and organ functions. Such functions will be described in the following chapters.

C O A R S E N I N G ← (down arrow)			Sense breathing Warmth Ego organization			R E F I N I N G ↑
			Saturn Jupiter Mars			
	Exhalation Water Ether organization	Venus Mercury Moon	Sun	Saturn Jupiter Mars	Inhalation Air Astral organization	
			Venus Mercury Moon			
			Earth Physical organization Metabolic breathing			

The harmonious and balanced interaction of the fourfold breathing process with the arterial and venous circulation process is the basis for sustained health.

At the same time the fourfold breathing process is in a different equilibrium in each organ of the human organization. It would be instructive to study each organ to find the particular balance in each one between the processes that have been described, both in health and illness.

Mineral remedies, which have a direct, healing effect on the four processes described, also extend their influence to the breathing and circulation process passing through all organs, because they affect the core of each process.

Furthermore the ego organization also directly participates through mineral therapy in the regulation of these processes. Its influence is then not merely organ-centred, but general and inclusive. Constitutional therapy with minerals treats the psychosomatic condition and the incarnation and excarnation process of the whole patient, beyond specific illness or pathological organ process. This constitutional treatment can then secondarily, through the harmonizing of the relationship of the members of man, heal the organic illness or disease.

If, instead, one wishes to exert a direct effect on one or more organ process, without involving the rest of the organism too strongly in the therapy, then plant medicines or organ preparations are usually indicated (e.g. Equisetum for kidney treatment).

We will take the first of these two paths and seek out those mineral substance processes in nature, which have an inner connection with the fourfold breathing process described. This will be done in the next chapter.

Following our description of the four aspects of the breathing process, we will now turn our attention to mineral substance processes in nature, the bearers of this fourfold breathing process. First we will examine, one by one, the four mineral substance processes, which relate to the activity of the fourfold breathing process. The mutual interrelationship of these four substance processes will then be studied, as well as their relationship to the threefold and fourfold organization and to the planetary metal processes within the human being.

The four substance processes are—

1 Phosphor: inhalation
2 Calcium carbonate: exhalation

3 Silica: sense breathing
4 Sulphur: metabolic breathing

1 Phosphor as the Driver of Inhalation

Within the human organism, phosphor is the 'driving motor for the inhalation of all inwardly directed breathing processes'. It thus manifests a polar process to that of calcium carbonate, which drives exhalation.[46]

The astral body, which receives the impulse for its activity through the phosphor process, brings air into the human organization via the lungs. In so doing it brings about 'inner oxidation processes' (combustion of carbon), and maintains the blood in a 'latent condition of fever'.[47] By regulating the intensity of organic combustion, it provides the basis for the ego's intervention; through the phosphor process (silica is also involved) the ego organization builds up a differentiated warmth organization, by intervening to regulate fever-inducing organic oxidation processes.

'The combustion of organic substance is the physiological basis of all will activity.'[48] The inner inhalation process activated by the astral body brings about the oxidation processes underpinning will activity. (Krebs cycle: transforming carbon into carbon dioxide and transforming adenosindiphosphate into adenosintriphosphate, an organ carrier of energy.)

Inhalation continues via arterial circulation into the organic activity of the metabolic–limb system.

The phosphor process strengthens the human being's lower ego organization in such a way that it can suppress the astral body's independent activity. This enables the lower, peripheral ego organization to take command of the astral body active in the metabolic–limb system.[49]

Phosphor must be carried by the ego organization via the blood, and thus prevented from its chemical release (except in trace amounts).[50] If the ego organization is too weak to prevent this, the physiological warmth process of the blood—a reflection within the physical body of the ego organization's activity—takes place autonomously, without the ego being able to participate. This results in peripheral inflammations, fever conditions and hyperaemia.

Brain activity is underpinned by a dynamic interaction of two polar tendencies, the inflammation tendency and the sclerosis tendency, as the physiological expression of the interaction in thinking between thought-forming activity (calcium carbonate, with functional involvement of silica) centred in the white substance of the brain (nerve-dendrites and Schwann cells) and will activity (phosphor, sulphur), centred in the grey substance of the brain (metabolic and nutritional activity of the nerve cell bodies).[51]

In the eye, as well as in all other sense organs, the functional relationship between silica (perception as reception) and phosphorus (perception as will activity) is of importance.[52]

Silica and phosphorus regulate the relationship of the ego organization and the astral body to one another.

Furthermore silica and phosphorus release the ego organization and the astral body from too strong a pathological connection within an organ; they regulate the way the ego organization and the astral body connect with and separate from the physical and etheric part of the organ.[53]

However, phosphorus influences the activity of the ego organization and astral body in the organs of the metabolic-limb system, while the silica process influences their activity within the organs of nerve-sense substance.

The phosphorus process (as does the silica process) involves the ego organization in the activities of mineralization and demineralization (polar Saturn processes), through its capacity to regulate the warmth process.

Phosphor reveals its relationship to the Jupiter process in its tendency to influence the liver's watery processes. If phosphor works too strongly, symptoms manifest of oedema, infectious hepatitis with jaundice or joint inflammations etc.[54]

The inner relationship of phosphor with the Mars process reveals itself among other things through processes of arterial circulation.

If the 'Mars-phosphorus process' is too strong hyperactivity, muscular hypertension, 'red' hypertension, tachycardia, polyglobulia, allergies, feverish conditions, pneumonia, cholecystitis with jaundice, manic states of excitement and agitation, and frenzy etc. can develop.

A weak 'Mars-phosphorus process' manifests as poor incarnation in the metabolic-limb system, for instance in the following symptoms: lack of will and motivation, lack of ability to make decisions etc. and on a physical level as muscular floppiness, low blood pressure, degenerative diseases.

The relationship of phosphor to the outer human planetary forces of Saturn, Jupiter and Mars can be convincingly elaborated with the help of Ala Selawry's book on metal-planet processes in man and nature.[55]

Phosphor supports the ego organization in such a way that it can 'overcome the opposition of the physical body'.[56]

2 Calcium Carbonicum (Conchae) as the Driver of Exhalation

Calcium carbonicum 'underlies and drives human exhalation'.[57] Through the calcium process, the ego organization and astral body participate in and regulate the exhalation process instigated by the etheric body.

But only a portion of the carbon dioxide forming in the lower organization is breathed out; a small part of it ascends into the head organization, and becomes the basis for the human capacity of thinking. The astral body takes hold of the carbon dioxide in a way that calls forth an activity of decomposition in the etheric and physical brain, which leads to the 'formation of thoughts'. Carbon dioxide works as 'breath poison', and creates a tendency to devitalize cells in the nervous system.[58]

The linking of calcium with carbon dioxide to form calcium carbonate enables the carbon dioxide process to enter into the working of the ego organization. By this means calcium can be directed towards 'bone formation' under the influence of nerve activity stimulated by the ego organization.[59]

Bone formation provides the organism with a solid basis for its shape and structure, while carbon, as bearer of the formative forces of the physical organization, is torn out of its solidity through the oxidation process and transformed to carbon dioxide in the lower organization. (This oxidation process is mediated by phosphor and sulphur). Through these two parts of the carbon process, the dissolution of bone substance and the reappearance of carbon in bone formation, 'the plasticity of form necessary for the physical body' arises.[60]

During embryonic development and in early childhood, the formative forces for our physical organization proceed from the nerve-sense system, but are then given over to the blood as formative forces of the organs.

Within the physical organization the calcium carbonate process mediates formative forces from the sphere of the three planetary processes of Moon, Mercury and Venus.[61]

These are 'formative forces for the organs of digestion and for protein substance'.[62]

(Silica, on the other hand, is the bearer of the polar opposite formative forces of the Saturn, Jupiter and Mars formative forces for the nerve-sense organs.)

The calcium carbonate process brings about the 'right relationship between the etheric body and the physical body within the nerve-sense organization.[63] This enables the physical, lightly mineralized brain to become a mirror for the thoughts awakened within the etheric body (e.g. concept-building as 'reflection process'). (Moon.)

The 'thought-forming process' itself has its physiological basis in the calcium carbonate building process.[64] A part of the calcium carbonate formed can be found as 'crystallization in the epiphysis region', while another part is directed into bone formation. This 'brain sand formation' is of importance for the development in the infant of the ability to form thoughts. The child becomes retarded if it is not present or insufficient.[65] The mineralized calcium carbonate in the brain enables the astral body to participate in thought formation. If it is lacking, the astral body cannot take hold of the brain organization because the brain's etheric and physical bodies remain too closely linked to one another, and so no mirroring can occur.

The Saturn mineralization process sustained by silica is significantly involved in the precipitation of calcium carbonate as mineral substance in the brain.

The Saturn process of light ether formation (see sense breathing), as the basis of thinking in the human being's upper sphere, is a devitalizing, cold process resulting in the precipitation of calcium carbonate from its dissolved state. This silica-borne Saturn process mineralizes the brain and encourages bone mineralization and bone formation.[66]

Phosphor and sulphur work in opposition to calcifying tendencies. They are warmth-bearing will substances that dissolve calcium carbonate formation through stimulating the blood-warmth process. As polar substances to calcium and silica they bring about a tendency to inflammation and demineralization.[67] Through both polar tendencies a continual depositing and dissolving of calcium carbonate takes place in the brain.[68] This is an expression of the interrelated working of thought formation and will activity in thinking (white and grey substance of the brain: conduction and nutrition).

Calcium carbonate used as medicine in high potency strengthens the formative functions of the Moon, Mercury and Venus processes. It encourages skull formation,[69] and also stimulates the mirroring, thought-forming function of the brain.

Through its fluid-expelling effect in the human being's metabolic system (originating in the head organization), the ego and astral body can be released from their pathological link with the water process in the metabolic organization, and then be available once more for activity in the nerve-sense system.[70] This can be indicated in phlegmatic, slowly responding, too dreamy and often lethargic patients with a tendency to water retention and lack of stamina.

On the other hand there can also be a tendency for calcium carbonate's head-forming forces to become too strong, so that the whole human being is in danger of becoming 'head'. In this case we see pallor, fear-fulness, anaemia, lithiasis, or the tendency for individual organs to become 'headlike'.[71] Such illnesses are caused by the formation of too much carbon dioxide from carbon, which makes the nerve-sense system work too excessively (Moon).

Higher potency calcium carbonate inhibits the development of carbon dioxide, so that, on the one hand, more carbon remains behind in the metabolic-limb organization and the blood; but on the other hand, less calcium carbonate is delivered into and active within the nerve-sense organization.[72]

But if too much carbon remains in the metabolic-limb organization, and too little calcium carbonate is active within the nerve-sense organ-ization, a tendency to fall back into the animal nature arises. This is expressed in increased irritability that can intensify to a tendency to hypocalcaemic conditions.[73] Insufficient breakdown of carbon is related in the lower organization to intestinal illnesses with diarrhoea, meteorism, burning pains etc. (Venus process.)

3 Silica (Quartz) as Bearer of Sense Breathing

The silica process underpins human sense activity.[74] Through sense activity a fine, 'crystallizing silica mesh or network' is integrated into us from above downwards. This internal quartz formation by the sense organization during sense perception enables us to open ourselves so wholly to the world of perceptions that we are in danger of completely losing ourselves in them. The tendency arises for us to become wholly sense organ. So as not to lose ourselves, therefore, we must dissolve the quartz network again in the very moment it forms. This occurs when we experience ourselves as 'I'.[75] The ego organization, with the help of the silica process, lives in this dynamic of opening to the sense world and returning to itself again through experiencing its bodily limits. To do this it needs to have mastery of the spirit of the silica process[76] in a way that enables it to regulate the polar process of forming the quartz network internally and dissolving the quartz again (Saturn). In silica's natural form in the outer world, as colloid and quartz crystal, we have a reflection of the dual ego organization process within the human being of crystal formation and dissolution.[77]

The silica process within the nerve-sense system (like the phosphor process within the metabolic-limb system), is a medium for the ego and astral body to take hold of the etheric and physical organizations. In the silica the nerve-sense process sustains the activity of the ego and astral body.[78] Silica enables the ego permeated by the astral body to partake in nerve activity.[79]

If the ego organization and the astral body have a pathological hold on the organism's nerve-sense substance, silica as a remedy can take over the pathological activity of the astral body and ego organization in the affected organ, releasing them from their involvement.[80] In this way the silica mineral's spirit and soul can enable the ego organization and astral body to learn to properly master and regulate the silica process in the organism.

'The silica process thus also regulates the interrelationship of the ego organization and the astral body, to bring about healthy sense activity'.[81]

If the astral body and ego intervene too strongly in the outer periphery of the nerve-sense organs and skin, these higher members become oversensitive to outer stimuli.[82] An over-predominance of the ego and astral body's activity in the sense organs and the skin prevents the ('sulphuric') nutrition process centred in the central lower organization from reaching the skin and sense organs. Silica in homoeopathic doses, or externally applied, can 'relieve the higher members of their excessive devitalizing activity in an organ, and thus open the way to nourishment processes'.[83]

At the same time silica also mediates ego activity in the head's nervous system, so that, under the ego organization's influence, the calcium carbonate formed from carbon dioxide is driven into bone formation. In this process calcium carbonate (and calcium phosphate) form the bone's mineralized substance. The formative impulse for the mineralization process and for the building of the boundary of bone substance (i.e. periosteum) and the rest of body tissue (i.e. skin) occurs through the Saturn force that is sustained by the silica process.[84]

Silica and calcium carbonate processes have a formative effect on individual organs and on the whole human form. Silica mediates the 'cosmic formative forces' of the outer planetary influences (Saturn, Jupiter and Mars), while calcium carbonate mediates the more 'earthly formative forces' of the closer, inner planetary influences. These latter are the formative forces of the 'Moon, Mercury and Venus'. Together they mediate the sun's formative forces.[85]

Silica and calcium carbonate mediate the formative forces of the whole solar system for individual organs and man's bodily organization. During embryo development (and also in the infant) these formative forces issue from the head, but later are passed to the blood, which then becomes both the bearer of the formative 'salty' and form-dissolving 'sulphuric' substance processes. The metallic 'mercury' processes mediate between them and maintain equilibrium.

Through the formative power of the silica process the ego organization can participate in the process of the formation of closing up the organism both within (the body) and without (nature), also a Saturn process. The ego organization thus has a limiting, forming and structuring effect, via the silica process, at the boundaries to both inner and outer worlds.

The ego forms an inner boundary at the bones (i.e. the periosteum), where the calcification process leads the living quality of calcium carbonate dissolved in the blood, into a lifeless state (crystalization).

The ego creates an outer boundary through silica by closing off the organism from the outer world at the skin, sense organs and the intestinal mucus membranes.[86]

In the sense-breathing process silica has a mediating but also limiting effect on the light ether, chemical ether and life ether of the macrocosm. In the nerve-sense organization, it halts the macrocosmic light ether (Saturn). In the rhythmic system, it draws a boundary for the influx of macrocosmic chemical ether (Jupiter). In the metabolic-limb system, it keeps the macrocosmic life ether separate from the lymph-forming and digestion process (Mars). Only the macrocosmic warmth ether is allowed unhindered passage through the organism.[87] This silica-mediated, limiting effect on the etheric forces of the outer planets corresponds to the forming of an individualized etheric organization.

The development of a differentiated warmth organism via the ego organization occurs in the equilibrium between the ego organization's silica-mineralizing and silica-dissolving activity within the nerve-sense system. In the metabolic-limb system, in contrast, a differentiated warmth organization is mediated by the phosphor process, and develops via the regulation of the blood warmth processes issuing from the peripheral, lower ego organization. In the silica and phosphor processes, the polar ego activity within the nerve-sense system and the metabolic-limb system meet one another in warmth regulation.

The macrocosmic etheric nutrition process of silica-based sense breathing encounters an inner creation of etheric forces that is stimulated through the nutrition and digestion process. The inner creation of etheric forces arises when the carbon made available through the nutrition process in the metabolic system (below the breathing) unites with oxygen to form carbon dioxide. The sulphur process sustains this carbon dioxide formation in the lower sphere. The carbon dioxide formation (oxidation) creates etheric forces, which penetrate and thereby strengthen the etheric body. This ether created within us draws the cosmic astral-etheric forces of sense breathing into the human organism, so that they can mediate formative forces for the development of organs.[88]

The silica and sulphur processes, bearers of cosmic and earthly nourishment, must be kept in equilibrium. If the sulphur process is too strong, the nutrition process of the metabolic system overwhelms the nerve-sense system. This can then, for instance, give rise to metabolic-product deposits in the organs of the nerve-sense organization.[89] If, on the other hand, the crystal-forming tendency of the nerve-sense organization (quartz formation) gains the upper hand, we see pronounced mineralization, with deposits, in the metabolic-limb organization (e.g. rheumatism, gout, kidney stones etc.).[90]

4 Sulphur as a Bearer of Metabolic Breathing

The sulphur process is a bearer of 'metabolic breathing'. As a 'sulphuric substance' it works primarily on the metabolic-limb system, which is the foundation for will activity.[91] In doing so it intervenes in the realm of the carbon process, stimulating digestion to greater activity. Via this intensification of digestion, sulphur also indirectly stimulates the activity of the heart and lungs (Mercury).[92]

Sulphur mediates between blood circulation and breathing, by transforming the 'digestive system orientated rhythm' (circulation) into a 'breathing orientated rhythm', which stimulates the exhalation process (Mercury).[93]

The sulphur process participates in the forming of venous blood in the lower organization. It mediates the connection between oxygen, breathed in with the help of the phosphor process and carried in arterial circulation (Mars), with carbon formed in the metabolic system, which produces the carbon dioxide of venous blood (Venus).[94]

It further supports the formation of protein-contained lymph plasma, which it is able to raise up into the sphere of the etheric body's activity

(Venus).[95] It renders carbon, the physical body's basic substance, more amenable to the etheric body's effect on it, and strengthens the astral body's involvement in the building of human protein in the lower organization (Moon, Mercury, Venus).

Besides its vitalizing intervention in lymph formation and digestion (Moon), sulphur regulates the absorption of lymph into venous blood formation and stimulates the cell-synthesis of the reticulo-endothelial system and white blood corpuscle formation (Mercury-Venus). Then, after the blood has become venous (Venus), sulphur leads venous circulation through carbon dioxide formation into carbon dioxide exhalation (Venus).

By inducing exhalation tendencies through a strengthening of the etheric body as against the astral body, it also encourages the capacity to sleep.

The sulphur process creates a close functional link between the etheric body and the physical body in the lower organization, strengthening the etheric body in its functionally restorative effect as opposed to the breaking-down dynamic of the astral body in the upper organization. At the same time, the astral body involved in up-building processes in the lower human sphere is stimulated to greater activity, corresponding to the 'night-phase of the astral body'.

4. THE PHILOSOPHER'S STONE

In nature, carbon (Carbo) manifests in three different modified forms: as coal, graphite and diamond.

Carbon manifests as diamond, the 'salt modification' originating from 'Old Sun'; as graphite, the 'mercury modification' originating from 'Old Moon'; and as coal, the 'sulphur modification', originating from late 'Lemurian times on earth'.[96]

	Diamond	**'SALT'**	**Old Sun**
Carbon	Graphite	**'MERCURY'**	**Old Moon**
	Coal	**'SULPHUR'**	**Earth**

Carbon as an element encompasses all three of these manifestations in *statu nascendi*.

Diamond is a special instance in the nature of carbon, one that arose on Old Sun. The transformation of carbon from its black, amorphous form into the crystallized, translucent diamond is a metaphor the sense world offers us for the future spiritual transformation of our physical embodiment. In the future man will come to have a physical body of a higher order and purity, consisting of a diamond-like material soft as wax.[97] He will then have taken the plant realm into his organism in such a way that he can accomplish the plant's assimilative processes within himself. The plant, after all, absorbs poisonous carbon dioxide for our sake, and exhales oxygen, using the carbon, which is left for structuring its own form.

In the future our breathing process will be transformed; the heart organ will enable blood rich in carbon dioxide to change into oxygen–rich arterial blood without taking in oxygen from our environment.[98] A part of the carbon dioxide necessary for this process will be obtained from calcium carbonate in bone as it dissolves. The metamorphosed 'carbon', which remains behind from this transforming process, will serve to build up the body and sustain our human form.

In this way a spiritual-physical body will form in us, similar to Christ's body of resurrection. This future spiritual-physical, immortal body, which has become plantlike at a higher level, will be one whose form no longer decomposes and is identical with the Philosopher's Stone known to the mystery stream of the alchemists.[99]

Physical death will thus lose all significance for human consciousness.[100]

Rosicrucian spiritual schooling taught[101] that the Philosopher's Stone is the highest level one can for the time being attain on a spiritual path. This stage of schooling and initiation is also described as 'Developing the Rhythm of Breath and Life'.

Transformation of the physical body into the Philosopher's Stone occurs through a particular regulation of the breathing process, which arises from constant and consistent meditative work (see above).

Rudolf Steiner describes how the human ego, with the help of this regulated breathing process, will gradually achieve complete mastery of its physical vessel.[102] An early step towards such mastery of the vegetative bodily functions, however, occurs by mastering circulation through breathing.

The balancing effect of the breathing process, which mediates physiologically between the nerve-sense system's physically-forming but catabolic activity and the life-enhancing, anabolic but form-dissolving activity of the metabolic-limb system, has a directly healing influence.

Carbon-alchemy of the human organism is, as we will see, linked to the 'fourfold breathing process' with its connection to the four substance processes quartz, sulphur, phosphor and calcarea carbonica.[103]

Carbon enables the human being's physical organization to maintain its specific form. The physical organization meshes with carbon structure.[104]

Carbon is the bearer of all formative forces, the bearer of the cosmic imaginations that form the physical body.

The human carbon process receives these body-structuring cosmic imaginations via the silica and calcarea carbonica processes. Silica mediates the cosmic formative forces of the outer planets (Saturn, Jupiter, Mars). Calcarea carbonica passes on to carbon and thus also to the physical organization the more earthly, inner planetary formative forces (Moon, Mercury and Venus).[105] Silica and calcarea carbonica form carbon, and thus the physical body.

Silica (Quartz)	Rhythmical balance (Gold)	Calcarea carbonica (Conchae)
Saturn, Jupiter, Mars	Sun	Venus, Mercury, Moon

In the plant, carbon itself regulates and balances the polar quality of the formative forces of silica and calcarea carbonica.

The form arising in the human being that is sustained by carbon must, in contrast to the plant, also be broken down. This takes place when carbon in man's lower sphere is transformed into carbon dioxide, and is mostly exhaled. As a result of the building and dissolution of the human form our human physical body receives the flexibility it needs. But part of the carbon dioxide is transformed into calcarea carbonica and, in skeleton formation, serves to create an underlying solid basis for our bodily form.[106]

Phosphor and sulphur processes play a decisive part in the dissolution of form through the formation of carbon dioxide from carbon. As a driver of inhalation,[107] the phosphor process conducts oxygen and nitrogen into the human organism as the activity of the astral body that is permeated by the ego organization,[108] and thus, by stimulating warmth processes, leads to inner combustion processes in the metabolic–limb system.[109] The actual formation of carbon dioxide from carbon is mediated through the sulphur process as an intracellular biochemical process. Through carbon's absorption into the carbon dioxide forming sulphur process, the ether-producing effect of carbon dioxide formation arises in the metabolic system with the aid of the oxidation-stimulating phosphor process.[110, 111]

That is to say: as the carbon arising in our lower sphere unites with vitalizing oxygen to form carbon dioxide, ether spreads at the boundary between exhalation and circulation, and permeates the whole organism. This ether, produced through carbon uniting with oxygen, takes up form-creating, astral–etheric forces that derive from the cosmic sense-nutrition process (silica).[112]

At the same time, part of the carbon—the bearer of form-creating forces—is transformed in this process into carbon dioxide. The carbon dioxide forming in our lower sphere is the foundation of an inner ether creation, which attracts cosmic formative forces from sense-breathing.

Carbon dioxide, created in the metabolic system, further stimulates, and exerts from the digestive organization a form-dissolving effect.[113] Here it works wholly in the service of the sulphur process that sustains metabolic breathing. The sulphur process, which conducts venous circulation into exhalation (Venus→Mercury)[114] and beyond, leads carbon dioxide upwards into the sphere of 'astral activity centred in the central nervous system', from where it is then expelled.[115] The etheric body, however, plays a decisive role in this exhalation process. Exhalation is driven by the calcium carbonate process,[116] which, with the help of the etheric and astral bodies, expels what is gaseous from the rhythmic system.

But part of the carbon dioxide is not exhaled, rising up instead into the nervous system. This carbon dioxide, which bears forces of devitalization and death in the head's nervous system, is the necessary physiological basis for thought formation.[117] On the one hand it enables the astral body to take hold of nerve substance,[118] and on the other hand it sustains the devitalizing effect of the physical brain's reflective function. Carbon dioxide, active in the upper sphere as effective basis for the thinking process, is also subject to the calcium carbonate process.[119] Thus the oyster-shell forming process (Conchae) can be seen as equivalent to human thought formation.[120] The calcium process not only enables the astral body to take hold of etheric-physical nerve-substance,[121] but also establishes the proper relationship between the etheric and the physical body in the head.[122] In this way the physical brain can become an appropriate mirroring instrument for cosmic imaginations present in the etheric body being transformed through the brain into earthly concepts and images. Part of the carbon dioxide unites in the nervous system with haemoglobin iron, and is led through the blood to exhalation.[123]

Another part of the carbon dioxide in the nervous system unites with serum calcium to form calcarea carbonica. Carbon dioxide in the form of calcium carbonate thereby becomes able to integrate itself into the activity of the central ego organization in the head. In this way the carbon dioxide in calcium carbonate is driven towards bone formation, with the help of head nerves in which the ego organization is active.[124] The functional calcium carbonate process, as the driver of warmth-etheric exhalation in the nervous system, prepares the ground for this by opening the way for the ego organization to take hold,[125] via the head nerves, of newly formed calcium carbonate substance in order to impel it towards bone formation. The central ego organization takes hold of calcarea carbonica substance via the head nerves and drives the mineralization of bones. The silica-sustained Saturn process regulates this process. The same process, however, is also present in the forming and depositing of calcareous crystalline substance in the pineal gland. This mineralization process enables the soul to grasp hold of thought-forming processes,[126] and works as a de-animalizing process.[127]

This is countered by bone-softening and decalcifying 'sulphuric processes' (sulphur, phosphorus) in the blood, which, via the process of brain decalcification, represent a fall-back to the animal level, with a general increase in hypersensitivity to outer stimuli (sense perceptions).

The calcarea carbonica process active in the nervous system is the bearer of the formative forces of the inner planets (Venus, Mercury, Moon). These forces, which during development in childhood are transferred from the nervous system to the blood, have the task of forming the protein substance (sulphur process) in the process of organ formation. The structuring antimony process occupies a mediating position between protein-creating sulphur and protein-structuring calcium carbonate processes.[128]

I have referred to regression to the animal level, with a general increase in the sensitivity of the nervous system (e.g. rachitic spastic tendencies) accompanied by reduction of calcium carbonate substance in the brain. A contrasting pathological regression into animality can also occur in the metabolic system, through absorption of carbon via nutrition. This is countered as it occurs by means of the complete breakdown of non-human carbon during digestion. Food-derived carbon must be destroyed in the intestines and rebuilt on the other side of the intestinal wall. This breakdown of non-human, food-derived carbon through digestion (Mars-phosphor process) and its recreation beyond the intestinal wall (Moon-sulphur process) is the precondition for overcoming regressive animal processes in our lower sphere. This enables the etheric body in our nerve-sense organization, stimulated through the cosmic light ether of 'sense-breathing', to create its own original light ether (Saturn-silica process).

If there is an inadequate breakdown of carbon in the metabolic system, relapse into the animal sphere manifests in symptoms such as burping, flatulence, putrid diarrhoea and heartburn, which we are familiar with from the homoeopathic pictures of Carbo, Sulphur and Phosphorus.

It should also be mentioned that the kidneys and urinary organs are involved in the breakdown of carbon. 'The calcium carbonate process in our nerve-sense system stimulates the excretion of bicarbonate from the blood via the urinary organs.' This can also be achieved through administering high-potency Carbo vegetabilis, which stimulates the kidney process.[129]

Before we can turn our attention to the transformation of carbon into diamond, we must first refer to the cyanide-building process (CN). This process, related to the limb system, in which carbon links with nitrogen to form cyanide (CN^-), competes with the carbon dioxide (CO_2) process that relates to exhalation and the head organization. Small amounts of cyan continually form within us. They have a close connection with human protein metabolism. If the ego organization is too weak to combine carbon and oxygen in forming carbon dioxide, too much cyanide forms. Such a disturbance arises when the cyanide-related sulphur process cannot be properly controlled by the ego organization. The consequence of such chronic cyanide intoxication is that too much calcium carbonate is deposited in the bones and blood vessels, so that they become brittle.[130]

The toxicological picture of acute cyanide poisoning arises through the combination of CN^- with trivalent iron (Fe^{+++}) in the enzymes responsible for oxygen utilization within the cell. As a result, oxygen from the arterial blood can no longer be absorbed within the cell, and this gives rise to intracellular hypoxia despite sufficient oxygen being available.

Acute cyanide intoxication can be treated in two different ways. The quicker way is through artificially induced met. haemoglobin formation, in which haemoglobin iron is led over from its bivalent to a trivalent condition. This trivalent haemoglobin iron then competes for cyan with the intracellular-respiration enzyme's iron, so that a first stage of detoxification occurs.

The second, slower way is through administering a salt, which is a sulphur compound. Ionized sulphur creates a new combination with the cyan-rhodanide (SNC^-), which is much less toxic and can be broken down by enzymes in the liver.[131]

It is extraordinarily interesting to note that the symptomatic manifestation of sulphur intoxication, for instance as caused by hydrogen sulphide or absorption of sulphur ions via the skin, is very similar to the symptoms of cyanide intoxication.[132]

It would go beyond the scope of this study to examine the mutual relationships between cyanide, carbon dioxide, oxygen and iron processes in muscular movement.[133]

The carbon process as the Philosopher's Stone and the gold process (Aurum) occupy the central position within our mineral system. These processes enable the ego organization to exert a balancing effect upon the primary, archetypal healing relationship between the rhythms of breathing and circulation.

When the ego organization establishes and sustains the rhythmic relationship between breathing and circulation (1:4–1:5), a dynamic equilibrium can develop from the rhythmic system between the 'salt' functions of the nerve-sense system and the 'sulphuric' functions of the metabolic system. This physiological equilibrium creates a condition in which the ego can exert a balancing effect on the astral body's threefold activity, by harmonizing thinking, feeling and willing. The fruit of this harmonization of thinking, feeling and willing is freedom and love,[134]

Calcium carbonate **Exhalation** 1 Ensouling of physical body 2 Mediation of inner planetary form processes 3 Formative forces of astral body in the physical body 4 Astral body takes hold of nerve substance 5 Regulation: etheric body ↔ physical body in the nerve-sense system 6 Brain as thought-reflecting instrument 7 Protein structuring			**'Salt'** **(Form)**			**Silica** **Sense-breathing** 1 Ego-permeation of physical body 2 Mediation of outer-planetary form processes 3 Formative forces of the ego in the physical body 4 Ego takes hold of the head nerves 5 Calcification of bones 6 Regulation: ego organization ↔ astral body in the nerve-sense system 7 Cosmic ether nourishment
Moon **Mercury** **Venus** (Metamorphosis)		'Sun–Mercury'	Ferrum sidereum	'Sun–Mercury'		**Saturn** **Jupiter** **Mars**
		Carbo vegetabilis	Arsenicum Album	Aurum metallicum		
		'Sun–Mercury'	Stibium metallicum	'Sun–Mercury'		
Sulphur **Metabolic breathing** 1 Inner planetary functions 2 Recreation and enlivening of physical body 3 Ether creation 4 Astral body takes hold of the metabolic-limb system 5 Earthly nourishment 6 Regulation: ether body ↔ physical body in the metabolic-limb system 7 Detoxification of the CN^- process; 8 Makes physical body more accessible to the ether body			**'Sulphur'** **(Force)**			**Phosphor** **Inhalation** 1 Outer planetary functions 2 Inhalation of O_2, N_2 3 Oxidation, warmth building 4 The ego organization takes hold of the metabolic-limb system 5 Destruction of food-derived carbon in the intestines 6 Regulation: ego organization ↔ astral body in the metabolic-limb system 7 Overcomes the physical organization's opposition to the ego's activity

which is identical with the 'gold-stream of the soul', the 'Golden Fleece' sought by alchemists.

This 'gold-stream of the soul', which was lost in previous human evolutionary epochs,[135] can work down upon the etheric and physical bodies and transform them.

Through preparation of the Philosopher's Stone, carbon—the nature of which is essentially earth-related—is transfigured into sunlike diamond.

The Philosopher's Stone, symbolized as wax-soft diamond, bears within it the future image of Earth evolution, of the time when the earth will spiritually unite once more with the moon and the sun.[136]

For us human beings this reunification also means, however, that we will transform moon-related forces of reproduction into a new, spiritually creative power. When this evolutionary stage is reached, man will become androgynous (mercurial), having elevated moon-related sexuality to the heart region, where it can then unite with the sun-nature of the 'I AM'.[137]

The physical body of man will be spiritualized into an immortal spiritual-physical body, which will be similar to the resurrected body of Christ and will become the basis for an eternal ego-consciousness beyond birth and death.[138]

A mineral therapy centred on the 'transformation of carbon' and the 'creation of gold' conceals 'Spirit Man' mysteries, which relate to evolutionary laws inherent in the ego, the physical body and the consciousness soul.

This study represents an attempt to understand and elaborate on these mysteries contained in the spiritual science of Rudolf Steiner and Ita Wegman, so as to render them fruitful for a constitutional therapeutic approach to chronic physical and mental illnesses.

	COSMIC (Saturn Jupiter Mars)	BALANCE (Sun)	TERRESTRIAL (Moon Mercury Venus)	
Nerve-sense system	Quartz (Si)		Conchae (Co)	'SALT'
Rhythmic system	Aurum met. (Au)	Ferrum sidereum (Fe) / Arsenicum album (As) / Stibium met. (Sb)	Carbo veg. (C)	'MERCURY'
Metabolic-limb system	Phosphor (P)		Sulphur (S)	'SULPHUR'
Members of man	Ego—Astral body	Astral body—Etheric body	Etheric body—Physical body	Regulation
Kingdoms of nature	Mineral	Plant	Animal	
Cognition Image building	Sense perception (SiO_2)	(Image)	Concept building ($CaCO_3$)	Past / Form / Rigidity
Feelings Emotions	(Sympathy) (Anger) (Embarrassment)	Courage and Balance and Love (Fe/As/Sb)	(Antipathy) (Fear) (Anxiety)	Metamorphosis / Rhythm / Development
Will activity	Motivation (P)	(Action)	Drive (S)	Future / Chaos / Flexibility
	Periphery Centripetal	BALANCE	Centre Centrifugal	
	Loss of identity		Loss of world relationship	

	COSMIC Saturn Jupiter Mars 'Peripheral'	BALANCE Sun	TERRESTRIAL Venus Mercury Moon 'Central'	
Nerve-sense system	Quartz (Si)		Conchae (Co)	'SALT'
Rhythmical system	Aurum met. (Au)	'Sun-Mercury process' $(Fe/As/Sb)$	Carbo veg. (Cv)	'MERCURY'
Metabolic-limb system	Phosphor (P)		Sulphur (S)	'SULPHUR'
Fourfold breathing process	Sense breathing (SiO_2)		Exhalation $(CaCO_2)$	
	Balance (Au)	Balance $(Fe/As/Sb)$	Balance (C)	
	Inhalation (P)		Metabolic breathing (S)	
Circulation	Arterial circulation	Capillary circulation	Venous circulation	

5. MERCURY AND THE UNITING OF OPPOSITES

As outlined before, there are three classes of substances within the mineral kingdom: Salt, Mercury, Sulphur. The threefoldness of the mineral kingdom, expressed in the three principles of Salt, Mercury and Sulphur, is related to a threefoldness of principles within the kingdom of plants (root, leaf, flower) and within the human being (nerve-sense system, rhythmical system and metabolic-limb system).[139]

This relationship between the three principles and the human organism and soul life in physiology and pathology has been once more summarized in the diagram at the end of this chapter.

We will now look at the three principles from the point of view of the Mercury principle.

The principle of Mercury is represented within the mineral kingdom by all metals (and by a few other substances like carbon). Although the metals bear within them all three principles, Salt, Mercury and Sulphur, the emphasis of their nature lies within the Mercury principle. The Mercury principle mediates between the crystalline nature of the salts and the inflammable nature of the sulphuric substances.

Mercury as a single and specific element is only one of the mercurial substances; because of its liquid nature, however, its ability to form and dissolve drops and its ability to build amalgam compounds with other metals it is a very representative one. (In the context of this work I use the term Mercury only for the principle and not for the metal, unless stated otherwise. Sulphur has equally a dual meaning as Sulphur principle—inflammable substance, storing light and warmth—and sulphur as a chemical element.)

As mercurial substances the metals have their main effect on the function and the consciousness associated with the inner organs. There is a relationship between metals and the organ functions/organ rhythms, and, in particular, a relationship with the rhythmical function of breathing and circulation, sleeping and waking, etc.

Metals, as a special group of minerals, support the ego organization to regulate the relationship between the astral and the etheric organization.

There are three metals that play a central role in their effect on the rhythmical system: Stibium metallicum, Ferrum sidereum and Arsenicum album.

Before we examine their indication we will first take a brief excursion into the field of Rosicrucian alchemy and anthroposophical cosmology.

The human Mercury principle is found within the rhythmical system (e.g. breathing and circulation). It is the archetypally healing principle within the human being, because it enables the ego organization to balance functional polarities like anabolism and catabolism, coarsening and refining, and—at the level of consciousness—willing and cognition.

Based on Rudolf Steiner's research, Walter Cloos describes the 'Double Mercury' of the Rosicrucian alchemists as a primary state of matter, in which the principles of Salt and Sulphur are completely dissolved within Mercury, and all three principles are not yet separated from each other. One finds this state of development in nature for example in unicellular organisms, in which sensory, rhythmical (breathing and circulation) and metabolic activity are not yet fully separated and differentiated.

According to Rosicrucian alchemy this 'Prima Materia' (English: Primary Matter) can still be found in the area between the physical and etheric of the human organization.[140] The author believes that aspects of this state of matter can still be found in the following three areas of the human organization:

1 Within the human blood, in which the ego, astral and etheric organizations balance and organize the warmth, air (oxygen, carbon dioxide and nitrogen) and corpuscular elements (blood cells) within a watery solution (serum). Within the blood, formative forces from the head organization (representing the Salt process and mediated by salt substances in solution, such as sodium, potassium, chlorine, carbonate etc.) as well as sulphuric life forces and substances (carriers of energy) from the metabolic system (such as proteins, fats, carbohydrates, organic phosphates etc.) are maintained in an equilibrium. ('Double Mercury')

2 Within human digestion, when foreign protein is broken down completely and freed from any foreign life process (the nutritional substance is brought into a state of chaos), before it is recreated as human individual protein within the metabolic organs and passed on to the blood. It then becomes the basis for the recreation of cells and organs.

3 During the process of conception and embryonic development, when male and female gonad cells unite, and tissues, organs and organ systems

form from the original zygote. During the process of conception, chromosomes and cell proteins are thrown into a state of chaos, which allows formative forces of the cosmos and of the incarnating spirit soul to influence the configuration of the inherited forces.

This primeval state of matter described as 'Prima Materia', Double Mercury, or 'chaotic world water' (Hebrew: *Tohoovabohoo*) leads back to an early stage of world evolution, named by Rudolf Steiner as the Lemurian time, in which the earth is a plantlike being and the human being not yet visible has an animal-like nature, and lives in the elements of warmth, air and water.

At this stage of Earth development, after the sun had departed from the earth and before the departure of the moon, the surrounding of the Lemurian earth environment is filled with a protein atmosphere and the earth has no solid centre.

Within this protein atmosphere the metals in their astral-etheric nature exert a certain influence on the Lemurian earth. The substance and the effect of these metals in astral-etheric form stems from the influence of the planets, which themselves have their origin during the Old Sun evolution.[141]

At this stage life exists in fast cycles of creation and destruction without any cellular forms. During this time the Stibium process plays a decisive role in organizing and structuring the living protein to create cells as smallest entities of life. The cells become the building stones for organs and organisms. This transformation of protein-bound life into cellular life cycles happens at this time, when the planet Mercury separates from the sun.

The Stibium process limits boundless growth by creating cells in a balance between anabolism and catabolism, dynamic (life) and form. This created cell organism has a mercurial nature in so far as it contains aspects of sensory and metabolic organization in still undifferentiated unity.[142]

Before Mercury and Venus separate from the sun, the separation of Mars from the sun takes place. The Mars planet's consistency is still astral-etheric, when it penetrates the Lemurian earth with its forces.[143] The Mars forces create the astral-etheric iron process within the Lemurian earth, which much later will condense to the solid iron as we know it today. At this time, when Mars exerts its strongest influence on earth, the astral-etheric iron process has a distinct influence on the development of the human organism still living invisibly in the elements of warmth, air and liquid; it creates the preconditions for the forming of red blood and of the breathing process. The human ego (self) will be empowered to incarnate within the not yet visible bodies of the human being as a result of preparing the creation of the red blood and the breathing process (as described above).

What has been outlined here about the influence of the astral–etheric Mars-iron process above finds its reflection in human embryonic development, in the forming of the embryonic circulation, the development of the placental circulation, the formation of blood and blood vessels within the embryo.[144]

Arsenicum helps the incarnation of the human astral body of the human being. Its effect on the cellular structures is that of organizing them in a way that allows the astral body to take effect from inside the cellular organization. This only becomes possible through inversion of the external world, the creation of an inner space separate from the outer space. This is the principle of organ formation, which in embryonic development manifests first when the gastrula of the human germ is formed. Organizing cells to build organs is an effect of the astral organization, using the Arsenicum and the Stibium process to mediate between the cells and the formative forces within the blood.

It has been stated above that the 'Double Mercury' is a state of primeval existence of matter, in which all three principles are in balance and *statu nascendi*. At this threshold of matter, which resembles past (and future) states of Earth development and matter, the Rosicrucian alchemist tried to conduct his experiments of transformation of impure metals into gold, and of the carbon process—which is a building block of primeval protein and carries the formative forces and the strength of the physical organization—into the Philosopher's Stone.

The transformation of impure metals into gold and the creation of the Philosopher's Stone aimed for a catharsis of the impure soul life (transforming non-precious metals into gold), a strengthening of the life forces and the creation of the immortal resurrection body (Philosopher's Stone).[145]

Rudolf Steiner describes how the 'Prima Materia' is created within the human body, whenever a harmonious relationship between thinking (cognition) and willing is created. Ferrum sidereum, Arsenicum album and Stibium metallicum as metals and mercurial substances help to bring about this balance and harmonious relationship between thinking and willing. All three metals help to regulate the functions of every cell and organ through the intracellular breathing process (inner and outer) and the circulation.

At the level of consciousness they help to develop courage (Ferrum sidereum) and reverence (Stibium metallicum) as a precondition for the development of freedom and love.

Arsenicum album represents the astral organization in its polar activity in anabolism (metabolic system) and catabolism (nerve-sense system). Arsenicum album, which regulates the day and night activity of the astral body, balances the effects of the Stibium process and the Ferrum sidereum process. The 'toxic and illness creating effect' of the astral arsenic process is transformed through the Stibium and the Ferrum sidereum process. At the level of consciousness this resembles the catharsis of the human astral organization.

Ferrum sidereum, Stibium metallicum and Arsenicum album help to carry the healing and transforming effect of the ego organization into the physical body, by harmonizing the polarities of thinking and willing and the polarity between nerve-sense activity and metabolic limb activity through their effect on breathing and circulation.

At the beginning of this chapter I outlined the three areas of the human organization in which we can find the mercurial state, which relates to the 'Prima Materia' and the 'Double Mercury':

1 The human blood in its relationship to breathing and circulation and to the principles of Salt and Sulphur.
2 The metabolic organization as the basis for nutrition, breaking down of food and recreation of individualized human body substance (protein).
3 The process of conception and embryonic development, where female and male gonad cells unite to create a new human organism.

I will now examine the function of Ferrum sidereum, Stibium metallicum and Arsenicum album within the human blood and the nutritional process.

The Ferrum sidereum Process (Meteoric Iron)

In the animal and human organism Ferrum (iron) is always bound to proteins (enzymes).

Ferrum is at work in all cells of the organism as an active component for those enzymes which are responsible for the intracellular breathing process (oxygen utilization and carbon dioxide elimination).

In the human blood iron is mainly bound to the haemoglobin of the erythrocytes,[146] but also circulates within the plasma or exists as ferritin iron (iron storage).

In the muscle metabolism iron plays an important role in facilitating the muscular activity.

Blood formation happens in the bone marrow (also in liver and spleen during foetal development). The vital stem cells of the erythrocytes lose their nucleus and with it their ability to reproduce.

The iron, which is bound within the haemoglobin, facilitates the process of oxygen intake (from outside through the lungs) and disposal (in the capillaries of the organs) as well as carbon dioxide intake and output. In the oxygen-rich arterial blood haemoglobin-iron carries mainly oxygen; in the carbon dioxide-rich blood iron carries mainly carbon dioxide. During foetal development, arterial and venous circulation are not as yet separate. This separation takes place at birth, starting with the first breath. At the same time breathing and nutrition separate too.

The red blood cells have a long maturation process, but within the bone marrow they are already subject to breaking down and deterioration processes. They lose their nucleus and their own metabolism and are then excreted into the peripheral bloodstream. From then on they have a lifetime of 120 days, but do not lose their function until the end of their life cycle. Old erythrocytes are eliminated within the liver and spleen. Bile is produced from the breaking down of haemoglobin within the liver (bile is very important for the proper digestion of food). Iron, which has been freed from the erythrocytes and is circulating in the serum, is absorbed by the liver and transformed into haemoglobin. The very active iron-metabolism follows a circadian rhythm (24 hours, the rhythm of the ego organization).

Iron influences the red blood cell's cycle of life and death. Within the circadian (24 hours) rhythm of the red blood a cosmic rhythm meets the rhythm of the human ego organization. The ego organization participates through iron in the formation and breaking-down of blood.

As mentioned above, a 120-days-old erythrocyte is still as functional as a young erythrocyte. This might be due to the life maintaining and conserving effect of the iron within the haemoglobin.

All body tissues and organs which have a high utilization rate of oxygen, like the nerve-brain tissues, the sensory organs and the epithelial cells of the kidney, are to a very high degree dependent on the life-preserving effect of iron and oxygen to compensate their devitalizing and catabolic tendency (nerve-sense dynamic). The healing effect of iron on these cells, tissues and organs is facilitated through the cell's own 'breathing enzymes'. Supplying the nerve cells with oxygen and utilizing this oxygen within the nerve cells is a function of the iron process, which extends its effect from the blood into the nerve-sense system.[147]

As mentioned above, the liver cells form bile as a by-product of the haemoglobin metabolism. The iron process regulates the bile production and secretion, as well as the excreting pancreas function. Through the iron process both the bile and the pancreas function become a tool of the ego and astral organization in the process of breaking down nutritional fats, carbohydrates and proteins. Nutritional proteins, fats and carbohydrates from the plant and animal kingdom need to be destroyed, so that their substance is freed from any alien etheric or astral forces. Only then can the human organism create its own individualized substances undisturbed, and the foreign astral and etheric forces are only needed to stimulate the body's own recreation of substance and etheric forces. Otherwise food would intoxicate the organism, and we would fall ill (allergies, food intoxication, inflammation tendencies etc.).

Foreign substance is not the only threat to human health, however, but also the body's own protein, which is created by the metabolic organs and leads to the regeneration of the organs and the blood. This protein-building process, facilitated through the sulphur process,[148] needs to be counteracted in the blood.

The life-creating protein process would put the human being at risk of losing his clear and alert consciousness; we would fall into a state of sleepiness and dreaminess (Lemurian consciousness), as well as fearfulness and powerlessness, if the iron process within the blood would not counteract it.[149]

The human being needs the deadening forces of the iron process within the haemoglobin to overcome the animalist tendencies of the protein-building process. Only with these deadening forces of the iron within the blood can the human ego partake in the earthly physical world with an alert consciousness.[150]

The balance between the life-creating protein-building process (sulphur) and the deadening iron process within the blood is particularly important during puberty, when the physiological birth of the astral body enhances the protein-building forces and the young person is at risk of falling ill[151] (anaemia, acne, inflammation tendencies, fatigue, anxiety, fear, illusions, depression, poor self-esteem, lack of self-confidence etc.).

The relationship between the protein-building process and the iron process is reflected in the building of protein-iron complexes, as in haemoglobin.

Human Blood	
Protein	**Iron**
Life	Death
Elevation	Gravity
Dreaminess	Alertness
Physical and etheric organization	Ego and astral organization

Iron helps the ego to overcome fearfulness and helps to develop courage within the rhythmical system (breathing and circulation).

In the nerve-sense system the iron process helps the ego to create an active thinking and an active perception, while within the metabolic-limb system it helps to develop a controlled and measured, but nevertheless strong-willed activity. The iron-binding protein (myoglobin) within the muscle cells mediates the latter process.

The iron process is not only introduced into the organism by means of ingestion, but also on a different pathway, through the skin and the sensory organs. Through these organs, the human organism absorbs the astral-etheric forces of the meteoric iron (cosmic iron) from the air and from the light. The sense organs absorb these astral-etheric forces of the cosmic iron and solidify these forces into elementary iron, which is connected with the body's own protein. The nutritional iron stimulates the process of sensory absorption and solidification.[152]

According to Rudolf Steiner the cosmic iron in light, air and earth stems from comets and meteorites, which in autumn are expelled by the sunspots. This indicates that iron remained in the sun after Mars separated from it. This cosmic iron-forming process is a contemporary one, opposite to the mineral iron compounds in the earth, which stem from the astral-etheric influence, exerted by Mars on earth in Lemurian times. As a very special Mars process the cosmic iron process has kept its close proximity to the sun. Rudolf Steiner describes the sun-originating cosmic iron process as being under the influence of Michael, the archangel inspiring the development of human freedom. Meteoric iron, which forms Michael's armour and weapons, is recreated within the human organization in the blood-forming process and, as an inner human process, is the foundation of the human being's ability to develop freedom.[153]

In childhood, Ferrum is absorbed into the organism, when the child is weaned and starts to eat earthly food. To develop his free will, the child needs to absorb iron through light, air and nutrition. The effect of the iron process in the child's development manifests first in the acquisition of his speech.[154]

Within the human blood the iron process counteracts, as outlined, the fear-creating and consciousness-paralysing forces of the protein-forming process.

By regulating the breathing process, the blood iron process keeps a balance between the life-creating arterial (oxygen rich) blood and the deadening, but consciousness-creating venous (carbon dioxide rich) blood. By keeping the balance, the iron process mediates, at the level of consciousness, between extremes of embarrassment and anxiety, helping to overcome the one-sided tendencies of both.

Within the muscular system the cosmic iron process unfolds its activity through myoglobin and helps to develop free movement between contraction and expansion. It helps to develop free will activity.

Within the nerve-sense system, the cosmic iron process carried by the oxygen-utilizing enzymes of the brain cells helps to activate human thinking by carrying will forces into the thinking and opens the thinking for moral intuitions (purposeful, creative ideas of the future).

In the support it provides for the development of freedom, the meteoric iron process shows its very close proximity to Silica, Aurum and Phosphorus, but also reaches further out into the area of the venous bloodstream with its connection to the inner planet processes of Venus, Mercury and Moon. It is able to do this because of its sun origin, and that is demonstrated by the fact that cobalt and nickel, two metallic siblings of iron, always accompany meteoric iron. Cobalt and nickel both show a number of characteristics of the metal copper.[155]

The sunlike quality of mediation between the forces of the inner and outer planets, as well as between the principles of Sulphur and Salt, underlines the truly mercurial (balancing and mediating) nature of meteoric iron.

Ferrum sidereum:

Nerve-sense system	Active thinking Intuition	Oxygen-utilizing enzymes in the nerve cells
Rhythmical system	Balance Courage	Oxygen/carbon dioxide Protein/iron
Metabolic-limb system	Strong and free will Measured activity	Bile and pancreas function Myoglobin

Stibium Metallicum (Antimony)

It has been described above that the function of the Stibium process in the evolution of the earth planet during the Lemurian times was to transform the protein process so that it could bear life into the cellular organism. Within the human organism today the Stibium process has similar functions. Stibium (antimony) works in close proximity to the Ferrum (iron) process as described above.

According to its nature and relationship to the human organism, Stibium has the following indications:

1 Stibium helps the patient, whose organism is unable to break down alien nutritional protein (due to a weak Ferrum sidereum process within the metabolism with weak pancreas and/or bile function), to integrate this alien protein into the human etheric organization and into the cellular metabolism.[156] Where Stibium cannot fulfil this function, the patient's organism is at risk of developing allergies, toxicity, or sustaining long-term damage to the metabolic organs like chronic inflammation and ulcerations (gastritis, enteritis, colitis, gastric and duodenal ulcers, irritable bowel syndrome, urticaria, acne, nephrotic syndrome etc.).

2 The Stibium (antimony) process plays a crucial part within the blood clotting process. 'Antimonizing (structuring) forces' within the blood work against 'albumenizing (protein-building) forces.'[157] Both processes need to be kept in a fine balance. If the protein building forces (sulphur, phosphor) overwhelm the structuring antimony forces, a haemorrhagic condition will result. Where the antimony forces overwhelm the protein-building process, a tendency to pathological blood clotting (thrombosis) will result.

3 The Stibium process is responsible for structuring protein so that the organs can be formed appropriately through the cosmic formative

forces within the astral and etheric organization. Stibium mediates between the astral and etheric body and integrates both harmoniously into the physical organs.[158] Ongoing worries, trauma or one-sided intellectual activity (enhancing the primarily catabolic and therefore destructive activity of the astral organization) can lead to deformation of the organ protein with the risk of organ destruction and/or pathological freeing of organic etheric forces, possibly leading to psychotic symptoms (such as hallucinations, delusions etc.). The pathological freeing of organ-bound etheric forces may enhance excarnation tendencies of the ego organization even further and schizophrenic-type conditions can develop. Stibium helps to reintegrate the astral and etheric body back into the organ and smoothes the way again for the ego organization to incarnate. Within anthroposophical medicine, Stibium is therefore one of the main remedies for the treatment and prevention of psychotic developments.[159]

4 Tendency to pathological softening of the consistency of the inner organs is due to a hypertrophic protein-building process. The organ swells up and loses its shape (e.g. chronic inflammation, hepatitis etc.).

5 Stibium harmonizes the relationship between the astral and etheric organization and therefore has a strengthening effect on the rhythmical system, especially the circulation. It is very useful in the treatment of cardiac arrhythmia but can also help if the organism is too sensitive to climate changes.[160]

6 The antimony process works particularly in the area between the breathing and sexual organization, i.e., within the digestive system and the circulation.

7 The antimony process helps neutralize outer influences on the skin that might lead to a predominantly catabolic and destructive activity within the skin, with devitalization of the skin expressed in the dry form of eczema and the formation of dandruffs, exfoliation, seborrhoea, ichthyosis, neurodermatitis etc. If the process progresses, highly inflamed forms of wet dermatitis can result. Eczemas caused by the above process can be treated with Stibium met. Antimony will harmonize the relationship between astral organization and etheric organization within the skin and will revitalize the skin through a better integration of the etheric in the physical organ.

8 Stibium has been used in the prevention of cancer. (See Dr Reimar Thetter, quote 161). This becomes understandable if one considers the carcinoma as chaos of form. The etheric organization has become too weak to integrate the pathological cell growth into the formative

principle of the organ and the organism. The cells lose their differ-
entiation and appear like embryonic cells. Stibium strengthens the
etheric and the astral organization, enabling it to better control and
integrate the growth of the tumour cells.

Within the human soul life, the Stibium process is related to the
development of reverence. Reverence in perception of the external
world opens the will for the influences of what is perceived (a similar
activity underlies the imitation process). The mental picture or image
(formative forces) can radiate down into the will organization and free the
will from its organic determination (protein-building process).

This is a cathartic process the ego can fulfil for the will: the ego
overcomes the animalistic nature of the will and can increasingly relate
harmoniously to the social environment.[161] Instincts, drives and desires
are transformed by the cathartic effect of mental images and a loving and
sociable activity can be developed.

On the other hand Stibium helps the ego to strengthen the capacity for
memory, the basis for the healthy development of one's own autonomous
personality. In this activity of ego-led memory, formative etheric forces
are freed from the metabolic organs and transformed into image-creating
memories within the nerve-sense system (brain).[162]

Stibium has a strong relationship to sulphur (etheric-physical protein-
building process) and calcium carbonicum (the bearer of formative forces
for the metabolic organs). As such it reveals its origin as having been
influenced by the combined and synthetic effect of the inner planets
(moon, Mercury and Venus).[163]

But the Stibium/antimony process reveals its mediating sun-mercurial
nature, inasmuch as it renders protein (sulphur and phosphor), and the
cells and organs, accessible to the formative forces of the ego (the human
Gestalt)—a silica process. It thereby not only mediates between the sulphur and the calcium carbonicum processes, but between the sulphur and
silica processes as well.

During embryonic and foetal development the Stibium process
connects the pre-earthly formative forces (silica, calcium carbonicum) of
the individuality from the past incarnation with the chaotic protein
(sulphur, phosphorus) of the dividing embryonic cells. The Stibium
process structures the protein within the dividing cells, so that the formative forces are able to take effect. This allows the development of a
human organism which can become the home for the incarnating ego.

Stibium metallicum

Nerve-sense system (Silica, calcarea carbonica)	Memory	Formative forces of the inner organs are freed and transformed into images	Brain Senses
Rhythmical system (Stibium metallicum)	Reverence	Balance between sympathy (ether body) and antipathy (astral body)	Clotting process (Balance) Circulation
Metabolic–limb system (Sulphur, phosphorus)	Social will (love)	Images transform the will (desires, drives and instincts) Inner structuring of organs	Forming organs from cellular protein

Arsenicum album

Arsenicum album is the oxide of arsenic, a chemical element and metal, which conducts electricity.

Arsenicum album is highly toxic and strongly affects the circulation and the digestion. The highly acute toxicological picture compares with that of cholera.

The slow intoxication leads to dryness and 'mummification' of the skin, severe sweating, poor circulation, cyanosis, gangrene, infarction of blood vessels with necrosis and bleeding. It further causes weight loss and anaemia. Hypersensitivity and hyposensitivity of many sensory organs have been reported.

The intoxication can be accompanied by feelings of severe anxiety, restlessness combined with a feeling of extreme weakness.[164]

Arsenicum album influences the protein metabolism, changing the nitrogen production. Further Arsenicum influences the glucose and lipid metabolism.

The remedy can have a biphasic effect, enhancing either anabolism or catabolism, depending on the individual constitution and the potency of the remedy. It therefore can treat polar conditions. It has a very strong affinity to the activity of the astral body in anabolism (metabolic system) and catabolism (nerve-sense system).[165] We can treat with Arsenicum symptoms of inflammation and sclerosis of all organs, but there is a particularly strong pathological affinity to the organs of the rhythmical system (breathing, circulation, sleep rhythm). Many of the other organ manifestations are the result of pathology of the circulation (vascular damage) and the breathing process (oxygenation, hypoxia, cyanosis).

At the level of consciousness, emotional symptoms, like severe anxiety, fear, sadness, despair, embarrassment, anger and guilt predominate—as one would expect from a remedy with such a strong affinity to the astral organization and the rhythmical system. And many mental symptoms, such as restlessness, compulsions and the tendency to control people and situations with a desire for perfectionism, are the result of, or a coping technique for, exposure to such strong emotions.[166]

Rudolf Steiner describes Arsenicum as a process related to the activity of the astral organization during the process of awakening.[167]

In the context of Levico spring water, an arsenic-containing spring water from a source in northern Italy, Rudolf Steiner describes how Arsenicum has a balancing effect on the polar iron and the copper substance within this water.[168]

Arsenicum has a balancing and mediating effect on the polarity of the astral organization activity within the metabolic-limb system dynamic (Stibium) and within the nerve-sense system dynamic (Ferrum sidereum).

Arsenicum album represents the astral organization's tendency to cause illness by losing the balance between anabolism and catabolism. The resulting pathology is mainly related to pathologic function within the rhythmical system. This tendency is reflected in the soul life by strong emotions, which tend either towards embarrassment and anger, or towards anxiety and fear.

Used as a remedy in connection with Stibium metallicum praeperatum and Ferrum sidereum, Arsenicum helps the ego contribute to the catharsis of the astral body by developing equilibrium between courage (Ferrum sidereum) and reverence (Stibium metallicum). Arsenicum helps to overcome the extreme manifestations of human emotions (astral body) and helps to prepare the development of freedom (courage) and love (reverence).

	Salt	Mercury	Sulphur
Substances, like	Silica Calcarea carbonica	Aurum metallicum Ferrum sidereum Arsenicum album Stibium metallicum Carbo vegetabilis	Phosphorus Sulphur
Quality	Substance crystallizes out from solution	Dissolving of salts or oils Falling drop	Tendency to burn by radiating warmth and light
Relationship to cosmos and earth	Earth building Centripetal	Mediating Balance	Cosmic Centrifugal
Plant kingdom	Root	Leaves	Flower
Human physical body	Nerve-sense system	Rhythmical system	Metabolic-limb system
Members of man	Etheric organization Physical organization	Astral organization Etheric organization	Ego organization Astral organization
Elements	Water Earth	Air Water	Fire Air
Function	Static Forming Densification	Rhythm (Breathing/Circulation) Solution Balancing	Dynamic Disintegration Refinement
Pathology	Sclerosis	Arrhythmias	Inflammation
Human consciousness	**Cognition** Perception Concept building Mental picturing	**Emotion** Sympathy Antipathy Empathy	**Will** Desire/Drive/Motive Force Deed
Soul-life	Conservatism, Persistence, Stability, Order, Stagnation Past	Balance, Evolution, Dynamic stability, Metamorphosis Presence between past and future	Progressiveness, Flexibility (change) Change, Chaos, Revolution Future
Virtues	Pure thinking Pure perception Moral intuition	Pure feelings Freedom Love	Pure will Ability to sacrifice Moral imagination
Potencies	LM 18 D 20–D 30	LM 12 D10–D15	LM 6 D 1–D 8
Characteristic of metals	Heaviness, Density, Hardness, Crystalline structure, Solid and characteristic form, Precious	Suppleness, Plasticity, Low melting point, Capable of forming alloys, Sheen	Vaporizes, Combustible, Colour, Smell
Kingdoms of nature	Minerals	Plants	Animals

6. GOLD AND THE PHILOSOPHER'S STONE

As sun metal, gold occupies a central position within our mineral system.[169] The gold process enables the ego organization to exert a balancing effect upon the primary, archetypal healing relationship between the rhythms of breathing and circulation. Gold is therefore especially effective as a remedy when these rhythms and their mutual relationship are disturbed, and when the cause of such disturbance does not lie in the nerve-sense or metabolic-limb systems but within the rhythmic system itself.[170]

When the ego organization via the gold process establishes and sustains the rhythmic relationship between breathing and circulation (1:4–1:5), a dynamic equilibrium can develop from the rhythmic system between the 'salt' functions of the nerve-sense system and the 'sulphuric' functions of the metabolic system.[171] This physiological equilibrium creates a condition in which the ego can exert an integrative effect on the astral body's threefold activity, by harmonizing thinking, feeling and willing. The fruit of this harmonization of thinking, feeling and willing is freedom and love.[172]

The harmonious relationship between thinking, feeling and willing which we need to attain anew is expressed in the 'salt', 'mercury' and 'sulphur' natures of gold and carbon. These three qualities of gold and carbon, which correspond with our threefold life of soul, are so solidly bound together in gold that it is difficult to separate them from one another. This is why gold is the most precious of the seven chief metals.[173]

But the gold process also mediates the balancing effect of the ego in relation to the soul functions and life processes issuing from the six planetary processes.[174] Here the ego-ruled gold process acts like the sun within the solar system, from which warmth, light, life and order radiate to the planets. In the human being the gold process can establish a harmonious equilibrium between the 'superior' and 'inferior' planetary forces of soul functions and life processes.

The 'Sun-Mercury process' mediates in the heart region between breathing and circulation, and balances between catabolic, cooling and formative 'salt' and anabolic processes, and inflammatory and form-dissolving 'sulphur' processes as well as inner ('I') and outer ('world') processes. Encompassing these great polarities in the human being is the

Aurum/Carbon–alchemy's central aim. This leads to the creation of 'Sun-Mercury', the 'higher spiritual gold process' within the human being. This physiological equilibrium creates a condition in which the ego can exert a cathartic effect on the astral body, by harmonizing thinking, feeling and willing.

What has here been outlined for the development of the human soul in its relationship to the substance processes accounts equally for physical illness and health.

Overly strong 'sulphur processes' (sulphur, phosphorus) will lead to inflammatory, feverish diseases; overly strong 'salt processes' (silica, calcium carbonicum) will lead to cold, chronic degenerative diseases, like stone forming and tumours. The 'Mercury process' (aurum metallicum and carbo vegetabilis) mediates between both. Pathology of the 'Mercury process' can lead to disturbances of physiological rhythms (such as breathing, circulation, sleep and waking etc.) or to rhythmical system organ illnesses (lungs, heart, blood vessels).

Dominance of the 'peripheral and centripetal forces' (silica, phosphorus) makes the body more susceptible to physical illnesses caused by environmental influences, like infections etc., while dominance of the 'central and centrifugal forces' (Calcium carbonicum, Sulphur) leads to illnesses that are rather caused by internal factors, like individual genetic pattern.

The Philosopher's Stone is formed, among other things, from the forces of carbon, calcarea carbonica and sulphur, supported by the planet processes of Mercury and Venus in their relationship to the Moon process.

The building of the gold process within the astral and etheric bodies is supported by aurum met., silica and phosphorus, which in turn are supported by the planetary processes of Saturn, Jupiter and Mars in their relationship to the Sun process.

The uniting of the gold process and the carbo process may lead to the development of the 'Sun-Mercury process', the archetypal balance of human forces as a basis for a dynamic state of spiritual, emotional, mental and physical health.

1 Calcarea Carbonica, Carbo Vegetabilis and Sulphur. The 'Positive Personality'. 'Memory and Love'

Calcarea carbonica, carbo vegetabilis and sulphur regulate the physiology of the CO_2 process within the human organism and therefore work on what Rudolf Steiner described as the 'blue (venous) blood tree', the 'tree of death' (CO_2), which is transformed into the 'tree of life' (C).[175]

Sulphur supports the creation of CO_2 out of nutritional carbon and creates life ether through this oxidation process within the metabolic system. Calcarea carbonica reduces the amount of CO_2 building within our organism, which allows carbon to be held back to build the future physical body of resurrection. Both processes balanced by the carbo process help the individuality to connect in love with the surrounding world and to overcome isolation and selfishness.

In this process, animalistic nature within the human organization and soul life (sulphur) can be overcome. By developing a loving and devotional relationship to the world around us (carbo), the human will becomes penetrated and transformed through the images gained in observation of the world (calcarea carbonica). These images, derived through sense perception and its processing, free the will increasingly from its organic dependency (animal nature based on instincts, drives and desires) and make the human will and actions a harmonious part of the social environment.

On the other hand the human being develops memories, which help the personality to sustain its ego-experience when facing the world and engaging with it. This remembering process works by lifting past experiences from the protein structure of the surface of the metabolic organs (sulphur) into the realm of nerve activity (calcarea carbonica), a process of memory leading towards consolidation of the personality.

Calcarea carbonica, carbo vegetabilis and Sulphur are indicated in patients who are too self-absorbed and too self-centred. They often lack interest for the environment and, due to often strong feelings of antipathy, find it difficult to develop devotion and love. As a consequence they often also lack perception, empathy and social adaptability.

In their social interactions they often seem odd and eccentric, because the will seems to be removed from any social perception.

They can show a tendency to be over-enthusiastic, hyperactive, too forceful and chaotic, defiant, rebellious, lacking in consideration and in self-knowledge, all signs of unformed and chaotic will activity (sulphur).

Or there can be a tendency to lethargy, laziness, inactivity, anxiety and worry about the future and their own health, as well as a paralysis of the will or a tendency to dyspraxia and/or apraxia, which indicates a predominance of the nerve-pole of the human organization (calcarea carbonica).

In both cases there can be a strong tendency to untidiness, although it can be a systematic kind of chaos.

People in need of calcarea carbonica, carbo vegetabilis and sulphur have the tendency to collect things and find it difficult to part themselves from old, now useless possessions. Personalities in need of these remedies are usually dominant and tend to form their environment ('positive personality').

The general physical and mental key symptoms of Calcarea carbonica, Carbo vegetabilis and Sulphur can be found in the table opposite.

Calcarea carbonica, carbo vegetabilis and sulphur as remedies in potentized form can help to overcome this one-sidedness of the character, helping to develop memory, self-confidence and love. This will lead to planned and measured activity, consideration, insight, tolerance, patience and self-knowledge.

2 Silica, Aurum metallicum and Phosphorus. The 'Negative Personality'. 'Initiative and Self-determination'

Silica and phosphorus regulate the physiology of the O_2 process within the human organism and therefore work on what Rudolf Steiner described as the 'red (arterial) blood tree', the 'tree of knowledge' (O_2), which is transformed into the faculty of freedom.[176]

Silica and Phosphorus regulate the intake of oxygen (inhalation) and the intensity of the oxygenation process, involving creation of life forces, energy and warmth.

On a mental level both processes allow courage and enthusiasm to develop. Courage and enthusiasm mediate between cognition (silica) and will activity (phosphorus) in four ways:

1 Will is carried into thinking, permitting the development of willed thinking, which can experience the reality of the future in the present through 'moral intuitions'.
2 The will is guided into the process of listening, permitting intuitive perception of the thoughts and the being of the other individuality.
3 Moral intuitions are transformed into ideals by feelings of enthusiasm, courage and love.
4 Ideals enter the sphere of the will and are transformed into 'moral imaginations'.

Moral imaginations build the new character of the individuality and have the tendency to become deeds.

	'The positive personality' 'Memory and love'		
Physiology	**Sulphur**	**Carbo vegetabilis**	**Calcarea carbonica**
	Metabolic activity	Vein formation Lung formation	Brain activity Mirror building
	Protein building	Breathing process (CO_2)	Exhalation Earthly nutrition (protein building) Carbon dioxide building process
		Venous circulation (CO_2)	
	Earthly nutrition	Balance between C and CO_2	Formative forces for the kidneys, bowels and genitals
Psychology	Sympathy, empathy, enthusiasm	Balance and harmony between cognition, emotion and will Harmony between 'I' and 'World'	Concept building Combination
	Will activity Wish Intention Resolution	Interest Empathy Love Reverence Memory	Antipathy Devotion
Pathology	'Positive personality' (forming environment) Too self-centred Too self-absorbed Lack of interest Lack of love Lazy Untidy Animalistic nature Loss of meaningful relationship with the world		
	Untidy Messy Too forceful Too chaotic Lack of consideration Lack of self-knowledge Defiance Rebellious	Over-enthusiastic/Lack of enthusiasm Flexibility/Rigidity Falling in Love/Rejection Self-confidence: too high/too low Lack of conscience/Over-scrupulous Mania-depression Over-enthusiasm/Lack of enthusiasm Fanatic/Doubter Greed for Life/Loathing of life Self-love/Self-condemnation Ruthlessness/Lack of courage Undisciplined/Self-disciplined	Too self-centred Egocentric Lack of perception Lack of empathy Lack of social adaptability Laziness Lethargy
Skill building	Planned and measured activity Consideration, Insight Tolerance Patience Self-knowledge	Will in harmony with environment Love Selflessness Benevolence (caritas) Sense of nature	Developing deep interest Empathy Compassion Social adaptability Devotion
	'LOVE'		

Silica, aurum metallicum and phosphorus are indicated in patients who are too sensitive towards any sense perception (photophobia, hyperacusia etc.). They tend to be too open in their social perception, oversensitive towards the strong emotions and actions of other people. They lack the ability to put up and maintain boundaries, and identify too strongly with their environment. As a result they often feel overwhelmed, drained in energy and emotionally exhausted. In their process of often (over-) sympathetic identification with other people, they can experience a feeling of confusion or loss of identity. Their good-hearted nature and their tendency to avoid conflict often makes them over-compliant and over-adaptable and puts them at risk of losing their independence. If attacked, insulted or offended, they find it difficult to defend themselves. People in need of silica, aurum metallicum and phosphorus are usually strongly influenced and formed by external life-circumstances, characteristics which Rudolf Steiner termed the 'negative personality'.

Despite the shared characteristics of phosphorus and silica, they are in many ways of polar opposite nature. People can be easily influenced by their environment, being gullible (phosphorus) or full of doubt, no longer daring to trust new experiences, holding on to past judgements as a means of protection (silica). They can be (over-) enthusiastic and (over-) joyful, and full of ever new interests (phosphorus) or melancholic and sad (Silica). The tendency of (over-) compliance (phosphorus) is complemented by the tendency to be stubborn, obstinate and rigid (Silica).

Patients in need of phosphorus have a tendency towards restlessness, hyperactivity and flightiness, whereas the silica-constitution shows signs of timidity, fear of failure and indecisiveness.

The general physical and mental key symptoms of silica, aurum met. and phosphorus can be found in the table on page 67.

Treating patients with silica, aurum metallicum and phosphorus helps them to establish an inner centre, to establish and maintain appropriate boundaries by helping to carry the activity and strength of the will (phosphorus) into the thinking process (silica). This inner activity of will-endowed thinking (aurum met.[177]) helps to develop independence and inner freedom.

On the other hand this treatment also helps to develop initiative, consistency, strength of will, courage and faithfulness by carrying ideas (silica) into the will (phosphorus).

This inner freedom becomes reality through the development of 'moral intuition', 'moral love' and 'moral imagination'.

	'The negative personality' 'Initiative and self-determination'		
Physiology	**Phosphorus**	**Aurum met.**	**Silica**
	Inhalation Oxygenation	Arteries formation Heart formation Uterus formation	Sense-organ building Sense-organ function Nerve function speech
	Spleen function	Heart function	Sensory function
	Liver function	Balance between breathing and circulation	Cosmic nutrition
	Limb movement Energy metabolism	Arterial circulation (O_2)	Formative forces for the senses, brain and larynx/lung
Psychology	Sympathy, empathy, enthusiasm	Balance and harmony between cognition, emotion and will Harmony between 'I' and 'World'	Faithfulness Courage
	Will Activity Intention Resolution	Self-determination Independence Courage Strength	Sense perception Contemplation Speech
Pathology		'Negative personality' (formed by life circumstances) Too open Lack of boundary Lack of self-protection Lack of independence Over-compliant Obsessively tidy Loss of identity	
	Lack of independence Lack of boundary Easily influenced Hypersensitivity Loss of identity Eagerness Over-enthusiastic Hyperactivity	Over-enthusiastic/Lack of enthusiasm Flexibility/Rigidity Falling in love/Rejection Self-confidence: too high/too low Lack of conscience/Over-scrupulous Mania-depression Over-enthusiasm/Lack of enthusiasm Fanatic/Doubter Greed for Life/Loathing of life Self-love/Self-condemnation Ruthlessness/Lack of courage Undisciplined/Self-disciplined Dictatorial/Servile Ailments from grief, anger, disappointed love, humiliation	Over-compliant Oversensitive Sadness Stubbornness Obsessively tidy Timidity Obstinacy Anticipation-anxiety Indecision Preoccupation
Skill building	Establishing an inner centre Establishing boundaries Inner activity Will-endowed thinking	Freedom Intuitive thinking Love of ideas (ideals) Moral fantasy Moral technique	Faithfulness Consistency Courage Self-confidence Strength of will
		'Freedom'	

3. *Ferrum Sidereum, Arsenicum Album and Stibium Metallicum. Balance Between the Positive and Negative Personality. Freedom and Love*

As metals, ferrum sidereum, arsenicum album and stibium metallicum represent the principle of 'Mercury' within the mineral kingdom. As minerals they stimulate the healing activity of the ego organization. The mercurial substances direct the ego activity to harmonize the relationship between the astral and etheric body, and therefore have a particular effect on the human feeling life, which swings between sympathy and antipathy.

The ferrum sidereum process helps to develop courage, to overcome fear and anxiety. Courage is a precondition for the development of freedom.

In its affinity to the arterial, oxygen-dominated part of breathing and circulation, ferrum sidereum supports the silica-aurum-phosphor qualities in the region of human feeling.

Feeling life mediates between cognition and will. The meteoric iron process develops courage in the feeling life, and activates the thinking by carrying the power of the will into the area of thinking. This will-activated thinking opens the mind for moral intuition. Moral intuition connects the true self of the human being with his future potential and creates new, spiritual motives for his deeds. This process frees the human being from being too formed and influenced by his environment.

On the other hand meteoric iron helps to transform intuitions into true imagination that forms and directs the will.

Rudolf Steiner described the meteoric iron process, which in the human being takes place in the forming and function of the iron-carrying haemoglobin, as an archetypal healing process, and as the physiological precondition for the development of freedom.

The stibium metallicum process helps to overcome feelings of hate and dislike for other people by developing a deep interest, care and love.

In its affinity to the venous, carbon dioxide dominated part of breathing and circulation, stibium metallicum supports the calcium carbonicum-carbo vegetabilis-sulphur in the region of human feeling.

The stibium-process (reverence) within the human being carries images as formative forces originating from the nerve-sense system into the will region of the metabolic-limb system.

The will can become enlightened by the images gained through observing the outside world with reverence. This enlightenment of the

Balance between the positive and the negative personality.
Freedom and Love

	Ferrum sidereum	Arsenicum album	Stibium metallicum
Physiology	Inhalation (O_2) Systole Arterial circulation	Rhythmical system Breathing Circulation Sleeping and waking	Exhalation (CO_2) Diastole Venous circulation
	Lungs Heart Blood vessels		
Psychology	Emotions		
	Antipathy	Equilibrium Harmony	Sympathy
	Intuitive thinking Courage Imaginative will	Balance	Memory Reverence Loving activity
Pathology	E.g.: arrhythmia, angina, asthma, carditis, pneumonia, TBC, sleeping disorder etc.		
	Emotional disorders: fear/anxiety/embarrassment/anger Mood swings Ambivalence		
	Overwhelming fear Violent anger Irritability Hypersensitivity	Obsessions and compulsions Paranoid delusions Anger with rage Severe states of anxiety and fear Extreme restlessness Tension Loss of sense of reality	Embarrassment Dislike of people Ailments from disappointed love Apathy Hyposensitivity
	Loss of self Lack of boundary	Loss of balance between self and world	Loss of world Lack of interest
Skill building	Freedom	Balance	Love
	Will into thinking	Balance between self and world Harmony	Memory
	Courage		Reverence
	Moral imagination	Self-restraint	Images into will

will gradually transforms and frees the will from its determination through the metabolism's animal-like life (instincts, drives and desires) and opens it towards a loving social relationship with the environment.

On the other hand stibium aids the process of remembering. Memory is a will activity, allowing forgotten experiences, which sank into the unconscious regions of the metabolism, to be raised into the region of consciousness once more. This ego-led activity of memory helps to consolidate the self-perception and autonomy at work in human consciousness, enabling it to maintain its continuity and alertness.

Arsenicum album mediates between the freedom–courage pole of the ferrum sidereum-process and the reverence–love pole of the stibium process, and unites both.

Anxiety, rigidity (obsessions and compulsions), embarrassment and hate can be overcome; and flexibility, adaptability, self-restraint and independence can be developed with the help of the arsenicum process.

Ferrum sidereum–arsenicum–stibium is indicated, if the human being suffers from a disorder primarily arising in the pathological relationship between the astral and etheric organizations, which can manifest itself in pathology of the rhythmical system and/or pathology within the human feeling life.

Both qualities of freedom and love are united in the ferrum sidereum–arsenicum album–stibium metallicum processes.

The Philosopher's Stone, symbolized as wax-soft diamond, bears within it the future image of Earth evolution, of the time when the earth will spiritually unite once more with the moon and the sun.[178] For us human beings this reunification also means, however, that we will transform the moon-related forces of reproduction into a new, spiritually creative power. When this evolutionary stage is reached, man will become androgynous (mercurial), having elevated moon-related sexuality to the heart region, where it can then unite with the sun-nature of the 'I AM'.[179]

Gold as the bearer of sun-forces and carbon as the representative of earth-forces unite in our heart region and, through the power of the human ego organization, help to metamorphose the human physical body into the body of resurrection.

A mineral therapy centred on carbon and gold conceals Spirit Man mysteries, which relate to evolutionary laws inherent in the ego, the physical body and the consciousness soul.

This study represents an attempt to understand and elaborate on these mysteries contained in the spiritual science of Rudolf Steiner and Ita

Wegman, so as to render them fruitful for a constitutional therapeutic approach to chronic physical and mental illnesses.

Although any spiritual development can mainly be achieved through life experience and a path of meditation and meditative experience, the experience, treatment and healing of illness prepare the described developments of freedom and love.

	Periphery Centripetal	Mediating (Rhythmically)	Centre Centrifugal	
NERVE-SENSE SYSTEM	Quartz (SiO_2)		Conchae ($CaCO_3$)	'SALT'
RHYTHMIC-SYSTEM	Aurum met. (Au)	Ferrum sider. (Fe) Arsenicum album (AsO_2) Stibium met. (Sb)	Carbo vegetabilis (Cv)	'MERCURY'
METABOLIC-LIMB SYSTEM	Phosphorus (P)		Sulphur (S)	'SULPHUR'
Cognition Image building	Sense perception (SiO_2)		Concept building ($CaCO_3$)	Past Form Rigidity
Feelings Emotions	(Sympathy) (Anger) (Embarrassment) (Au)	Courage (Fe) Self-restraint (As) Love (Sb)	(Antipathy) (Fear) (Anxiety) (Cv)	Metamorphosis Rhythm Development
Will activity	Instinct Drive Desire (P)		Wish Intention Resolution (S)	Future Chaos Flexibility
	Loss of identity	Lost balance between 'I' and 'Self'	Loss of relationship with the world	

	'Peripheral'	'Central'	
NERVE–SENSE SYSTEM	Quartz (SiO_2)	Conchae ($CaCO_3$)	**'SALT'**
RHYTHMIC SYSTEM	Aurum met. (Au)	Carbo veget. (Cv)	**'MERCURY'**
METABOLIC–LIMB SYSTEM	Phosphorus (P)	Sulphur (S)	**'SULPHUR'**
Sensing Breathing Circulation Nutrition	Sense perception	Brain function	
	Cosmic nutrition	Exhalation (CO_2)	
	(SiO_2)	($CaCO_3$)	
	Arterial circulation	Venous circulation	
	(Au)	(Cv)	
	Inhalation (O_2, N_2)	Metabolic activity	
	Limb movement	Earthly nutrition	
	(P)	(S)	

7. PRACTICAL APPLICATIONS

The LM potencies

As outlined in the previous chapters of this study, the effect of potentized mineral remedies on the human constitution will now be considered. It has been stated that mineral remedies in homoeopathic preparations have a specific effect on the relationship between the ego organization and the lower members of man. In strengthening the ego organization's power to work on transforming the astral body, ether body and physical body, homoeopathic mineral treatment strongly supports the development of the consciousness soul. (See chapters 1, 2, 3.) This effect can be further enhanced through the choice of the method of the potentization.

LM potencies (LM6, LM12 and LM18) of mineral remedies have shown particular efficacy in the treatment of chronic physical and mental illnesses. Compared with high potencies (C30–C200–C1000–XM– . . .) they have a very good safety record and can be safely used even in weakened patients with terminal conditions (like cancer or burned-out schizophrenia). LM potencies of mineral remedies are usually more effective in the treatment of chronic conditions than D or C potencies of mineral remedies.

The author of this study, like some other anthroposophical physicians, has used LM potencies (LM6,12,18) in the constitutional treatment of chronic illnesses, and they have become an invaluable tool in the treatment of these conditions. Besides their impressive efficiency and good safety record, it is reasonably easy to handle them, to monitor their effect and to adapt them to the patient's individual response to the homoeopathic treatment (slowness to respond or strong initial aggravation reaction).

LM potencies can be used alongside allopathic medications (like antipsychotic, anti-depressive and anti-epileptic drugs) without interfering with patients' metabolism, and I have seen marked improvements of chronic conditions even in patients who have been on a long-term drug regime. Any other anthroposophical or potentized (metal, mineral, plant or animal) remedies (between D1 and D30) can complement LM potencies without any disturbing interaction.

LM6, LM12 and LM18 are the potencies on the LM scale I recommend using for constitutional treatments with potentized mineral remedies and for the use of nosodes (see below).

The deep-acting and long-lasting somatic and psychological effect of LM potencies are often experienced, and can be better comprehended by looking at the process of potentizing.

To make a LM6 potency from a mineral, one will have first to produce a C3 trituration (3 triturating steps of 1:99).
1 part of the C3 trituration is dissolved in 99 parts of ethanol 95%—LM1.
1 drop of this solution impregnates the surface of 500 little pills (of which 500 pills weigh 1 gram)—LM2. (The impregnated pills are placed on filter paper to dry.)
1 pill of LM2 is dissolved in 100 drops of ethanol 95% and seccussed 100 times—LM3
1 drop of solution LM3 impregnates 100 pills, which are then air dried—LM4.
This process of potentizing in 2 half-steps (solid–liquid–solid) is repeated until LM18 is produced.

(LM stands, not quite correctly, for $L = 50/M = 1000 = 50,000$, which is the dilution factor within one LM step. In reality, we are dealing with 2 half-steps of 1:100 (solid to liquid) × 1:500 (liquid to solid), which only mathematically results in a factor of 1:50,000.)

The LM6 potency is not a high potency. In mathematical terms it is a dilution of 10^{-33} (comparable with a D30 potency). This degree of dilution is achieved in rhythmical steps of potentizing starting with 3 C steps (1:99) and with 6 LM steps. From a different point of view the 6 LM steps are 12 LM half-steps, amounting to 15 steps of potentizing. The 6, 9 or 15 steps of potentizing, which lead to a dilution of $1:10^{30}$ (D30), indicate that the LM6 potency might show the quality of a medium high potency, possibly encompassing the effects comparable with a D6, D9, D15 or D30. Equally LM12 and LM18 show the effect of a medium high potency.

Practical experience with the LM6, LM12 and LM18 potencies showed the following:

The LM6 of a mineral remedy works primarily on the metabolic-limb system and from there into the other systems.

The LM12 of a mineral remedy works primarily on the rhythmical system (breathing/circulation) and from there into the other systems.

The LM18 of a mineral remedy works primarily on the nerve-sense system and from there into the other systems.

The following case shows the effect of Argentum met. LM6 in strengthening the metabolic-limb system. Treatment was for a deeply exhausted and depressed 25-year-old medical student who had been suffering from a malignant gonad tumour; the testes had been removed and the patient received some radiotherapy and was in a state of mental depression and physical exhaustion for two months afterwards. Treated with Argentum met. praep. LM 6 he recovered from the depression and exhaustion completely within five weeks. (Alternatively I would have used Argentum met. praep. D6.)

In my medical practice I have been using the mineral remedies in LM6, 12 and 18 potencies for conditions that originate in one of the systems of human threefoldness.

I have been using mineral remedies in LM potency for the treatment of chronic schizophrenic patients with remaining positive and negative symptoms despite long-term treatment with different psychotropic agents in combination. Treating patients with these potentized anthroposophical remedies over several months, my therapist colleagues and I have observed considerable improvement of positive and negative symptoms in some of them, although they still continued with their allopathic drug regime. In many cases it was possible to reduce allopathic medication with the cooperation of a psychiatrist without any adverse effect on the patient. In most of the patients we have seen an improvement in their social skills and motivation. They had greater ability to make and sustain contact with other people and to sustain a job. There was also an improvement of mood and reduction of anxiety in most hospitalized patients with mental health problems, and even in residents with moderate to severe learning disabilities. Although the treatment of patients with chronic conditions takes time to be effective, I have never seen such long-lasting and deep healing effects with remedies in potencies between D1 and D30 as I have observed with LM potencies.

An explanation for the nature of the effect of LM potencies on the human constitution can be gained if one looks at the pharmacological process itself. In producing the LM potency, the medium/carrier of the potentized force is changed rhythmically between liquid and solid or between impregnation, evaporation and dissolving. (*Solve et coagula* is one of the major underlying principles of this potentizing process and shows a particular relationship to the alchemical 'salt process' that can remind us of conditions in the Lemurian times of earth development, after the separation of the moon from the earth, when solid minerals first came into existence.)

By changing the medium rhythmically from alcohol (liquid) to lactose pillules (solid) and back, spiritual forces of the original substance are freed which seem to be particularly effective in the region between the human etheric (liquid) and physical (solid) body or in the region between life and death. In chronic physical or mental illness the relationship between the ether body and physical body within one or more organs is disturbed. In the hallucinatory condition symptomatic of psychosis, for example, life forces are pathologically freed from the organs and take effect within the soul life in a way that disturbs mental health. On the other hand, in chronic physical illnesses like cancer, part of the individual etheric body is too deeply bound into the physical organ and leads to its destruction. The embryonic quality of low-differentiated tumour tissue gives us an idea of the strong connection between etheric and physical forces within the tumour.

Mineral remedies in D potencies do not seem to have as deep an effect on the balancing and healing of the relationship between the etheric and the physical body as LM potencies appear to. Nevertheless, mineral remedies in LM potencies also show a clear effect in strengthening ego activity within the other members of man, for example in patients where the improvement of active short and long-term memory, self-perception and self-determination has been observed.

The treatment with these remedies in LM potencies further seems to have an effect on the catharsis of the astral body. Conflicts within the unconscious life of the soul are often activated within days of treatment and surface in dreams that can be remembered better than usual on waking and during the daytime. Extreme emotions like anxiety, fear, shyness, embarrassment, anger, hate and so on are moderated and can come under the patient's control.

Long-term applications of mineral remedies in LM potency often seem to have a moderating effect on one-sided temperament, for example easing the extreme expressions of a choleric or melancholic temperament. Patients in whom life forces seem to be weakened, for instance in post viral syndromes or in earlier stages of terminal cancer, often seem to improve to some extent.

Symptoms of obsessive-compulsive disorder have been reduced, which indicates a partial freeing of parts of the ether body from the hardening physical forces of the lungs.

To sum up, my experience with mineral remedies in LM potency make them seem a useful tool in the treatment of chronic physical and mental illness, due to their enhanced effect on the ego organization and the relationship between the patient's etheric and physical body.

Indications for the use of mineral remedies in LM potencies
Constitutional treatment of psychosomatic disorders, psychological disorders, chronic physical illness or chronic mental illness.

The Use of Nosodes

As this study centres on the use of mineral remedies for the constitutional treatment of chronic physical, emotional and mental illnesses, this section is kept rather short. Nevertheless the nosodes play an important role, as they complement the effect of mineral remedies in an important way.

Nosodes are potentized preparations originating from human diseased tissue. As human products in potentized form, they have a direct transforming effect on the physical organization, which is the carrier of the individual inherited forces. Starting from the physical organization they extend their effect into transformation of the etheric and astral body. The direction of their action is opposite to that of the minerals, which work transforming the ego organization downwards to the lower members of man.

They are entirely safe remedies, because they are inactivated, highly diluted and potentized. Nosodes are used for the treatment of deep-seated inherited constitutional problems. Nosodes have been shown to complement treatment with mineral remedies where the latter fail to show the expected reaction or effect. This happens when either the etheric organization is too weak to respond or the physical organization is too rigid and hardened, and the etheric and astral organization are entrapped within the hardened physical organization. We might find this condition in some genetic syndromes or inherited diseases, as well as after long-term use of allopathic drugs.

In this regard they act as preparation for the efficacy of mineral remedies to follow, and are comparable with the reaction enhancing effect of Carbo vegetabilis and Sulphur, but on a deeper and more immediate level (the physical organization is directly affected by the nosodes). In this regard they work transforming the physical model and the forces of inheritance, like childhood diseases do during the first seven years of life.

The nosode used in this context for the transformation and healing of the forces of inheritance is:

Tuberculinum.

This preparation is made from a culture of mycobacterium tuberculosum, originally grown in a human being.

Tuberculinum is one of the major nosodes for the treatment of autistic spectrum disorder. Tuberculinum helps with exposure anxiety, hyper-sensitivity, restlessness, lack of adaptability and ritualistic behaviour.

There have been many decades of therapeutic experience in the use of this and other classic nosodes for the treatment of learning difficulties, emotional and behavioural problems, mental health problems and genetic disorders.

Nosodes are further often useful to prepare and intensify the treatment with other more specific constitutional remedies, such as the above outlined minerals. After the use of a nosode, a well chosen remedy might start to work, although it had failed to be effective prior to the use of the nosode.

Tuberculinum affects the rhythmical system, which mediates between nerve-sense-activity (salt) and metabolic-limb-activity (sulphur) as well as between peripheral organization (Saturn, Jupiter, Mars) and the central organization (Venus, Mercury and Moon).

The lung organ, which is most affected by Tuberculosis, is the central earth organ and has a distinct relationship to the carbon process.

Tuberculinum stimulates and strengthens the life forces of the organism and can therefore be indicated in states of exhaustion, weakness and/or lack of reaction to well chosen constitutional remedies.

Tuberculinum helps transform the inheritance forces within the physical organization (as childhood diseases do!).

Tuberculinum mediates between inflammation and sclerosis tendencies. Both tendencies are characteristic manifestations of this disease (fever, inflammation, granuloma, and calcification)

The homoeopathic proving picture of Tuberculinum overlaps essentially with the proving picture of all the above outlined mineral remedies and prepares their use.

Tuberculinum can be used whenever the physical organization is so hardened, that it overpowers the enlivening effect of the etheric organization. This is the case in chronic conditions, in which the organism responds unsatisfactorily to a well-chosen constitutional remedy. As such, Tuberculinum has a similar catalytic effect to Sulphur (and Carbo), but on a deeper level, as Tuberculinum is able to target the hardening of the physical organization more directly.

Tuberculinum is therefore part of the constitutional remedy compositions for the treatment of chronic ill health.

Treating Chronic Physical and/or Mental Conditions with Mineral Remedies and Nosodes in LM Potency

Indication

Constitutional treatment of psychosomatic disorders, psychological disorders, chronic physical illness or chronic mental illness.

This constitutional treatment is not directed at a specific illness and its symptoms, but treats the underlying psychosomatic pattern, stimulating the self-healing and self-regulating powers of the patient suffering from a chronic illness. It thereby contributes indirectly to improvement in symptoms of ill health.

The remedies can, if necessary, be applied in conjunction with other specific allopathic, potentized or anthroposophical medication.

The remedies stimulate the harmonizing of the soul forces of cognition, emotion and will power, and support the development of the power of self-determination, independence and a loving relationship towards the social environment.

Extreme emotions such as anxiety, fear, shyness, embarrassment, anger, hate, sadness and despair are moderated and come under the control of the patient. The remedies often have a mood-stabilizing effect and help to develop courage, love and equilibrium.

The regenerating power of the patient's organism can be activated. Patients whose life forces are weakened as a result of long-term chronic illness often recover their lost energies and overcome feelings of weakness, fatigue and lethargy.

The immune system can be boosted and a tendency to recurrent infections improved.

A balance between inflammatory, form-disintegrating and sclerotic, hardening tendencies is stimulated. Anabolic (dissolving) and catabolic (coarsening) forces within the physical body are balanced.

Application

Beside using some of the outlined substances as single remedies in LM potency, the use of the following three remedy-compositions has proven an effective and gentle intervention for many patients in the treatment of chronic conditions:

1 **Carbo comp T12 (O.P. Weleda UK)**
   (Calcarea carbonica LM18/Carbo vegetabilis LM12/
   Sulphur LM6/Tuberculinum LM12 aa)
2 **Aurum comp T12 (O.P. Weleda UK)**
   (Silica LM18/Aurum met. prep. LM12/Phosphorus LM6/
   Tuberculinum LM12 aa)
3 **Arsenicum comp T12 (O.P. Weleda UK)**
   (Ferrum sidereum LM18/Arsenicum album LM12/Stibium met.
   prep. LM6/Tuberculinum LM12 aa)

Duration of treatment

Treatment can be continued under the physician's two to three-monthly supervision as long as an improvement of the symptoms and of the patient's general well-being continues.

Stopping the treatment too early after improvement can cause the reappearance of symptoms in milder form and warrants a reintroduction of the remedy.

A change of the remedy composition is indicated if the improvement comes to a halt, some of the old symptoms reappear, or if new symptoms develop.

Side effects:

First aggravation

During the initial phase of treatment (usually within 3 weeks after introducing the remedies), a temporary aggravation of the patient's symptoms of ill health can frequently be observed, which usually completely disappears within days or a few weeks after the introduction of the remedy and tends to make place for considerable improvement of the patient's condition thereafter. It can still be necessary to counteract too intensive an initial aggravation by introducing a break in treatment for several days, and/or by reducing the frequency of application for a few weeks thereafter, until the organism has adapted to the new treatment.

Anamnestic reaction

During treatment, the reappearance of year-old symptoms is not uncommon. These symptoms of past diseases are experienced and worked through in a mild and very accelerated way. This 'anamnestic reaction', which is well known as a healing reaction in classical homeopathy (Hering's law), indicates that treatment does not suppress symptoms but heals by working through past constitutional pathology. This is underlined by observations that a by-product of treatment is the strengthening of ego activity and a maturation of the patient's personality.

The recurrence of old symptoms as an 'anamnestic reaction' therefore needs to be understood as a healing reaction.

The experienced physician has to discriminate between genuine aggravation (progressive illness), 'initial aggravation reaction' and 'anamnestic reaction', because each of these situations will require a different course of action.

Interaction

The above outlined remedies in LM potency can be complemented by allopathic medication and/or other remedies from anthroposophical medicine, such as potentized metals, plants or organ preparations or, where necessary, with allopathic drugs. No adverse interactions with other medications have so far been reported.

Intercurrent illnesses

Intercurrent illnesses like viral or bacterial infections can be treated with other medications without having to discontinue the constitutional treatment with the LM potency of mineral substances, although in some cases it might be advisable to introduce a short break.

APPENDIX TO CHAPTER 2
RUDOLF STEINER'S COMMENTS ON THE MINERAL KINGDOM

1. The Efficacy of Mineral Remedies: From a Lecture of 8 December 1908 (GA 107)*

... A remedy derived from the mineral realm works initially on the human being's physical body. Now what purpose is there in someone administering a mineral remedy to his physical body? Please be clear that we are not talking here about any kind of plant-derived remedies, but of purely mineral ones, consisting of metals, salts etc. Imagine that we take some mineral remedy or other—something very remarkable then becomes apparent to clairvoyant perception. Clairvoyant vision always has the capacity, you see, to divert its attention away from something, from the human being's whole physical body in fact. Then one observes the etheric body, astral body and ego-aura. Through a strongly 'negative' focus of attention you can suggest away the physical body. Now when someone has taken a mineral remedy, you can divert your attention away from everything else, and focus it solely upon the mineral or metal that he has ingested. You suggest away the bones, muscles, blood etc. and focus attention only on the particular mineral substance permeating his organism. Then something very remarkable appears to clairvoyant awareness: this mineral substance disperses itself in very fine solution throughout the organism, thus assuming the shape of the human being. You therefore see before you a human form, a human phantom as it were, consisting of this substance. Let us assume that someone takes a dose of antimony—then you will see before you the human form composed of finely dispersed antimony; and the same occurs with every mineral remedy that we ingest. We create a new human being within us, con-sisting of a particular mineral substance; we integrate it into us. What is the purpose and sense in this?

It has the following purpose: if you left someone who needs some-thing like this as he was—in other words if you did not give him the

---

* English edition: *Study of Man* (Rudolf Steiner Press, 1966).

remedy he really needs—his astral body, because of certain damaging energies and forces it contains, would affect his etheric body and this in turn would affect his physical body in a harmful, destructive way. Now, though, you have permeated his physical body with a 'double', which means that the physical body does not respond to the influences exerted by the astral body. Imagine a runner bean plant: if you give it a stake to climb up it winds itself around it and no longer grows the way the breezes blow. This double, composed of a substance someone ingests, is a similar kind of prop for him. It trains the physical body to itself and withdraws it from astral and etheric influences. By doing this you make the physical nature of the human being independent of his astral and etheric bodies. That is the effect of a mineral remedy. But you will immediately see the negative aspect of this, for it does also have a very negative aspect. When you artificially remove the physical body from its integration with the other bodies, you also, at the same time, weaken the influence of astral and etheric bodies on the physical, thus making the physical body more independent. The more you administer such remedies, the more the influences exerted by astral and etheric bodies fade, so that the physical body becomes hardened and independent in itself, and thus subject to its own separate laws. Just think what people do who dose themselves throughout life on various mineral remedies. Someone who gradually ingests many such mineral remedies comes to bear the phantom of these minerals within himself; he's full of such mineral remedies, and they constrain the physical body, as though within four walls. What influence can his astral and etheric bodies still exert on him? Such a person drags his physical body around with him and is fairly powerless against it. If such a person, who has dosed himself in this way over a long period, then tries to get a different kind of treatment—which aims to address his mental and emotional state through working on the finer bodies—he will find that he has become more or less inaccessible for finer mental and emotional influences. He has made his physical body independent and thus removed its potential for receiving what might occur in the finer bodies, for letting such finer influences work down into it. And this occurs chiefly through the fact that he has so many phantoms within him, which do not work harmoniously together; one pulls him one way, the other another way. Once such a person has rendered himself unable to access his soul-spirit aspects in this way, he need not be surprised to find that a course of more rarefied treatment, addressing the spiritual in man, has little success in his case. Thus, when it is a question of treating a person's emotional and mental state, you should always consider what sort of person you are treating. If the patient has rendered his astral or etheric bodies powerless by making the physical body independent, then it is very difficult to help such a person with a cure that addresses the spirit.

So you can understand now how mineral substances affect the human being. They create doubles within him, which preserve his physical body and withdraw it from the potentially harmful influences of his astral or etheric body. Almost all medicines today are based on this principle, for today's materialistic medicine is unaware of man's finer bodies, and tries only to address his physical body in some way or other ...

Author's comment
This passage describes the effects of failure to digest non-potentized mineral substances or remedies. The above description also holds good, in my opinion, for so-called food additives such as laboratory processed vitamins and multi-minerals, as well as for refined nutritional products, such as salt, sugar and chemical additives. It also accounts for allopathic medication. Although allopathic medications and food additives can often be very helpful in the treatment of many conditions in the hand of an experienced doctor or therapist, they still have the tendency to alienate the physical body from the influence of man's higher members. Thus they can become obstacles in the process of spiritualizing the physical organization.

Mineral remedies in sufficiently high potencies are transformed through their manufacturing process into 'spirit-like qualities' (cosmic world-ego qualities of the mineral from the Thrones; see above) and therefore have the opposite effect on the human constitution from non-potentized and 'not fully digestible' minerals. Potentized substances strengthen the ego organization and soften the physical organization, thus counteracting the above-described effects of unpotentized minerals and supporting the physical organization's transformation and spiritualization.

2. From a Lecture Given in Dornach on 30 March 1920 (GA 312)

What we have separated more or less last from ourselves is what we must also take back soonest into ourselves in the healing process ... we separated ourselves from the actual mineral kingdom later than from the plant kingdom, and we must be clear that seeking a connection to the plant world alone is a one-sided endeavour. Yet the plant kingdom does remain instructive for us nevertheless, because when the plant heals it does not do so merely through its plant nature, but through the fact that it also contains the mineral kingdom within itself ... But we must be aware that the plant is actually reworking anew a part of what is present in the mineral kingdom, and that what it thus reworks and processes does not have such healing properties as what has not yet been worked upon.

3. *Rudolf Steiner and Ita Wegman:* Fundamentals of Therapy *(GA 27), Dornach 1925, Chapter XVII,* 'Knowledge of substances as the basis for knowledge of medicaments' *

Medicines derived from the plant kingdom will be able to heal a disturbed relationship between etheric and astral activity. But such remedies will not be effective when something in the human being's physical, etheric and astral organization is disturbed in its interaction with the ego organization. The ego organization must direct its activity to processes that tend towards mineralization.

This is why one only needs mineral remedies to tackle such conditions. In order to understand the particular healing effect of a mineral substance, we need to examine a substance to see how much it can be broken down, for a mineral substance introduced externally must be broken down in the organism and rebuilt in a new form through the organism's own forces. Healing consists of this breaking down and newly reforming. The result of this must be, more or less, that the organism's lack of inner activity is taken over by the activity of the remedy introduced into it.

4. *Rudolf Steiner,* The Temple Legend,[†] *Extract from Lecture 13 (Third Lecture, Berlin 29 May 1905): Concerning the Lost Temple and How it is to be Restored*

... For what in general is the task of the human being in his earthly evolution? He has to raise the present three bodies with which he is endowed to a higher stage. Thus, he must raise his physical body to a

---

* Current English edition: *Extending Practical Medicine* (Rudolf Steiner Press, 1996).
† (Rudolf Steiner Press, 1997.)

higher realm and likewise his etheric and astral bodies. This development is incumbent upon humanity. That is the real sense of it: to transform our three bodies into the three higher members of the whole divine plan of creation (Manas, Budhi, Atma).

There is another kingdom above that which man has immediately and physically around him. But to which kingdom does man in his physical nature belong? At the present stage of his evolution, he belongs with his physical nature to the mineral kingdom. Physical, chemical and mineral laws hold sway over man's physical body. Yet even as far as his spiritual nature is concerned, he belongs to the mineral kingdom, since he understands through his intellect only what is mineral. Life, as such, he is only gradually learning to comprehend. Precisely for this reason, official science disowns life, being still at that stage of development in which it can only grasp the dead, the mineral. Science is in the process of learning to understand this in very intricate detail. Hence it understands the human body only in so far as it is a dead, mineral thing. It treats the human body basically as something dead with which one works, as if with a substance in a chemical laboratory. Other substances are introduced [into the body], in the same way that substances are poured into a retort. Even when the doctor, who nowadays is brought up entirely on mineral science, sets about working on the human body, it is as though the latter were only an artificial product.

Hence we are dealing with man's body at the stage of the mineral kingdom in two ways: man has acquired reality in the mineral kingdom through having a physical body, and with his intellect is only able to grasp facts relating to the mineral kingdom.

This is a necessary transitional stage for man. However, when man no longer relies only on the intellect but also upon intuition and spiritual powers, we will then be aware we are moving into a future in which our dead mineral body will work towards becoming one that is alive. And our science must lead the way, must prepare for what has to happen with the bodily essence in the future. In the near future, it must itself develop into something which has life in itself, recognize the life inherent in the earth for what it is. For in a deeper sense it is true that man's thoughts prepare the future. As an old Indian aphorism rightly says: What you think today, that you will be tomorrow.

The very being of the world springs out of living thought, not from dead matter. Outward matter is a consequence of living thought, just as ice is a consequence of water; the material world is, as it were, frozen thoughts.

We must dissolve it back again into its higher elements, because we grasp life in thought. If we are able to lead the mineral up into life, if we transform [it into] the thoughts of the whole of human nature, then we will have succeeded; our science will have become a science of the living and not of dead matter. We shall raise thereby the lowest principle [of man]—at first in our understanding and later also in reality—into the next sphere. And thus we shall raise each member of man's nature—the etheric and the astral included—one stage higher.

What man formerly used to be we call, in theosophical terminology, the three elementary kingdoms. These preceded the mineral kingdom in which we live today, that is, the kingdom to which our science restricts itself, and in which our physical body lives. The three elementary kingdoms are bygone stages [of evolution]. The three higher kingdoms—the plant kingdom, the animal kingdom and the human kingdom—which will evolve out of the mineral kingdom, are as yet only at a rudimentary stage.

The lowest principle in man (the physical body) must indeed still pass through these three kingdoms, just as it is at present passing through the mineral kingdom. Just as today man lives in the mineral kingdom with his physical nature, so in the future he will live in the plant kingdom, and then rise to still higher kingdoms. Today with our physical nature we are in a transitional stage between the mineral and plant kingdoms, with our etheric nature in transition from the plant kingdom to the animal kingdom, and our astral nature in transition from the animal kingdom to the human kingdom. And finally, we extend beyond the three kingdoms into the divine kingdom, with that part which we have in the sphere of wisdom, where we extend in our own nature beyond the astral . . .

. . . Be clear from now on about the respective positions of plant, animal and man. The plant is the precise counterpart of man. There is a very deep and significant meaning in our conceiving the plant as the exact counterpart of man, and man as the inverse of plant nature. Outer science does not concern itself with such matters; it takes things as they present themselves to the outer senses. Science connected with theosophy, however, considers the meaning of things in their connection with all the rest of evolution. For, as Goethe says, each thing must be seen only as a parable.

The plant has its roots in the earth and unfolds its leaves and blooms to the sun. At present the sun has in itself the force, which was once united with the earth. The sun has of course separated itself from our earth. Thus the entire sun forces are something with which our earth was at one time permeated; the sun forces then lived in the earth. Today the plant is still searching for those times when the sun forces were still united with the earth, by exposing its flowering system to those forces. The sun forces are the [same as those which work as] etheric forces in the plants. By presenting its reproductive organs to the sun, the plant shows its deep affinity with it; its reproductive principle is in an occult way linked with the sun forces. The head of the plant [the root], which is embedded in the darkness of the earth, is on the other hand similarly akin to the earth. Earth and sun are the two polar opposites in evolution.

Man is the inverse of the plant; the plant has its generative organs turned towards the sun and its head pointing downwards. With man it is exactly the opposite; he carries his head on high, orientated towards the higher worlds in order to receive the spirit—his generative organs are directed downwards. The animal stands half-way between plant and man. It has made a half-turn, forming, so to speak, a crosspiece to the line of direction of both plant and man. The animal carries its backbone horizontally, thus cutting across the line formed by plant and man to make a cross. Imagine to yourselves the plant kingdom growing downwards, the human kingdom upwards, and the animal kingdom thus horizontally; then you have formed the cross from the plant, animal and human kingdoms.

That is the symbol of the cross.

It represents the three kingdoms of life, into which man has to enter. The plant, animal and human kingdoms are the next three material kingdoms [to be entered by man]. The whole evolves out of the mineral kingdom; this is the basis today. The animal kingdom forms a kind of dam between the plant and human kingdoms, and the plant is a kind of mirror image of man. This ties up with human life—what lives in man physically—finding its closest kinship with what lives in the plant ... The sun is the bearer of the life forces, and the plant is what grows in response to the sun forces. And man must unite what lives in the plant with his own life forces. Thus his foodstuffs are, occultly, the same as the plant. The animal kingdom acts as a dam, a drawing back, thereby interposing itself crosswise against the development process, in order to begin a new flow.

Man and plant, while set against each other, are mutually akin; whereas the animal—and all that comes to expression in the astral body is the animal—is a crossing of the two principles of life. The human etheric body will provide the basis, at a higher stage, for the immortal man, who will no longer be subject to death. The etheric body at present still dissolves with the death of the human being. But the more man perfects and purifies himself from within, the nearer will he get to permanence, the less will he perish. Every labour undertaken for the etheric body contributes towards man's immortality. In this sense it is true that man will gain more mastery of immortality the more evolution takes place naturally, the more it is directed towards the forces of life—which does not mean towards animal sexuality and passion.

Animalism is a current which breaks across human life; it was retardation, necessary for a turning-point in the stream of life. Man had to combine with animalism for a while, because this turning-point had to take place. But he must free himself from it again and return again to the stream of life . . .

5. From the History and Contents of the First Section of the Esoteric School 1904–1914. Letters, Documents and Lectures.★ *Leipzig, 13 October 1906 (GA 265)*

One can even acquire a fine perception for the lifeless mineral kingdom. The minerals have a group soul on the Devachan plane, just as the animals possess a group soul on the astral plane. The souls of the minerals live in Devachan. Therefore they are not available to man. As the fly when it walks over our hand is unaware that there is a soul within it, so have men no notion that stones have souls.

If stones possess souls, then you will also be able to understand how a moral understanding of them can arise. A human or animal body has desires, passions and driving-impulses. The body of a plant no longer contains any passions but it still has a driving force. The body of the stone has neither desires, nor driving force, therefore it sets an ideal for man in that our impulses must become spiritualized. And in the far distant future of mankind that will be accomplished; man will possess bodies without desires and impulses. One day man will be like a diamond; he will no longer have inner impulses, but such things will then be outwardly under control.

The mineral already displays such chastity today—it is matter without desire. The occult pupil must already cultivate this desirelessness at the present day. In this sense the stone stands higher than animal, plant or man. An ancient Rosicrucian saying states: I have placed and hidden the

---

★ (Anthroposophic Press, 1998.)

eternal creator word in the stones; chaste and modest they hold it in the depths of physical existence.

If one can raise such perception of the stones into spiritual experience, one will become clairvoyant in the highest regions of Devachan.

6. *From a Lecture in Stuttgart, 14 June 1921*

Now man in his temporal existence between birth and death is so constituted that he carries forces within him that continually kill him. Those are the forces which make him solid and firm, which are involved in the building up of the skeleton and, in their morbid aspect, lead to sclerosis, gout, diabetes and so forth. These are the forces which man has within him, which I should like to call the solidifying forces. That is the one thing. The other system of forces man has within him is the one that continually rejuvenates him. It is the power system that is especially typified when one succumbs to pleurisy, feverishness and everything that occurs together with a high temperature. From the anthroposophical point of view I have called the solidifying forces ahrimanic and the forces leading to fever, which are warmth forces, I have called luciferic. Both of these forces have to be kept in continual balance within the human being. If they are not kept in balance they lead mankind in body, soul and spirit to some kind of fatal extreme. If the feverish forces are not continually kept in check by the solidifying (salt-forming) forces [and vice versa], then the person will inevitably develop sclerosis or get a temperature. If a person develops only his powers of understanding and has a leaning towards intellectuality he will fall a prey to Ahriman. If he develops only his fiery element of desires and emotions, he will succumb to Lucifer. Thus man is always placed between two polarities and has to hold the balance.

But just think how difficult it is to hold the balance. The pendulum, which ought to be in balance, always tends to swing to one side or the other. There are three tendencies in man: the tendency towards balance, that towards warmth and that towards solidification. The human being has to stay upright, so that one can typify man symbolically as a being who has to continually struggle to maintain his upright position in the face of the three forces, which are always threatening his life . . .

The threefold human organism and the mineral kingdom

	Cognition			Feeling			Will		
	Perception	Image	Concept forming	Sympathy	Equilibrium Harmony	Antipathy	Instinct Drive Desire	Motive	Wish Intention Resolution
Physical systems	Nerve-sense system ▼			Rhythmical system ▲▼			Metabolic-limb system ▲		
Organs	Sense organs		Brain	Lungs (Breathing)	Heart, Blood vessels (Circulation)		Organs of metabolism		Muscles
Function	Sensory function Sense organs		Mirror building Brain function	Inhalation Oxygenation	Exhalation Carbon dioxide		Nutrition Anabolism		Limb activity
Minerals	SALT			MERCURY			SULPHUR		
Physical systemic functions	Forming, Cooling, Mineralizing (lithiasis), Devitalizing (Death), Slowing down, Forming, Differentiating			Breathing and circulation Inhalation (O_2)–Exhalation (CO_2) Systole–diastole Circadian rhythms Sleeping and waking			Nutrition, Regeneration, Reproduction, Vitalization, Anabolism, Warming, Dissolving form, Acceleration, Movement		
Physical pathology	Sclerosis, Cancer, Chronicity, Stone formation, Gout, Diabetes			Arrhythmia, Angina, Asthma, Carditis, Pneumonia, TBC, Sleeping Disorder			Inflammation, Fever, Acuity (E.g. Meningitis, Pneumonia)		

	▼	▲ ▼	▲
Psycho-pathology	**Cognition:** Stubbornness, Obsessive thoughts, Fixation, Repetition, Dogmatism, Rigidity, Preoccupation, Slow processing **Feeling:** Sadness, Grief, Fear, Anxiety, Apathy, Flatness, Disgust, Autism **Will:** Passivity, Compulsion, Paralysis, Slowness, Repetition	**Affective Disorder:** Feelings and mood overwhelm, Cognition and will, Mania/depression, Mood swings, Ambivalence, Loss of sense-self, a) too high, b) too low, Loss of sense of reality, Dreamlike state	**Cognition:** Gullibility, Delusions, Flightiness, Hallucination, Confusion, Fast processing **Feeling:** Overjoyed, Anger, Shame, Euphoria, Agitation, Aggression, Emotionality **Will:** Hyperactivity, Chaos, Rage, Violence, Hectic
Healing and social skills	Strength of will, Adaptability, Flexibility, Activity, Courage, Empowerment, Self-confidence	Freedom and love, Will into thinking, Images into will, Independence, Devotion	Wisdom, Consideration, Insights, Patience, Consistency, Planned and measured activity

APPENDIX TO CHAPTER 4

1. From the Lecture of 21 May 1907 in Munich★

What is the meaning of the two pillars of the Rosicrucians? If we are to explain the meaning of the two pillars, which we have before us here, we must take our start from the Golden Legend. This is as follows.

When Seth, the son of Adam—who took the place of Abel—was sufficiently mature, he was vouchsafed a glimpse of Paradise. He was allowed to pass by the angel with the fiery sword and enter the place from which mankind had been banished. Seth saw something very special there. He saw how the two trees, that of Life and that of Knowledge, were entwined together. From the two entwined trees Seth received three seeds, which he took with him and placed in the mouth of his father Adam after his death. A mighty tree then grew out of the grave of Adam. This tree then appeared to people with psychic vision as though shining with a fiery glow and this glowing light twined together, for those who could see it, to form the letters J B, the initial letters of two words, which I am not allowed to pronounce here, but of which the meaning is: 'I am He who was; I am He who is; I am He who will be.' This tree divided into three branches. Seth took some wood from it, which was used in various ways during world evolution. A rod was made from it, which, according to legend, was the magical wand of Moses. It was the very same wood from which the beams of Solomon's Temple were made. They remained there for as long as mankind could still understand the ancient secrets. Then the wood was thrown into a pool, from which at certain times lame and blind people could receive healing. After having been retrieved from there it was formed into the bridge across which Our Saviour trod as He went on his way towards the Cross. And according to the Legend, the wood of this tree, which had grown up out of Adam's mouth from the seeds planted therein from the entwined trees of Life and of Knowledge, was formed into the very Cross upon which Our Saviour hung.

This legend has a deeply symbolic meaning. Think for a moment of that transformation, which the pupil has to contemplate when he takes

---

★ Translated by John Wood.

the fourth step in the Rosicrucian training, the production of the Philosopher's Stone. We recollect that this entails a particular way of dealing with our red blood. Let us consider the significance of this red blood, not only on account of Goethe's allusion to it, 'Blood is a very special fluid', but because occultism of all ages has taught us this. As red blood exists it is the result of breathing oxygen. We can only briefly allude to that. When we are referred in the Legend and in the Bible to that very important moment of Seth's renewed entrance into Paradise, we must call to mind the reason for mankind's expulsion therefrom. Man was expelled from Paradise—his old condition of rest in the lap of the higher spiritual world—through what is hinted at in the Bible as the parallel physical accompaniment to his descent. Whoever wishes to understand the Bible must learn to take it literally. It is said: 'God breathed into man's nostrils the breath of life, and man became a living soul'. That which is pictured here, as inhalation of the breath of life, was a process stretching over millions of years. What does it mean?

There have been times during the creation of physical man in which he did not possess lungs, so that the inhalation of oxygen could not then take place. There were times in which man lived more or less in the liquid element and during which he had an organ something like air bladders, from which the lungs later developed. These former air bladders were transformed into lungs and we can follow their transformation. When we do so this process is revealed as what is described in the Bible as God breathing into man's nostrils the breath of life and man becoming a living soul. With this inhaling of breath, the creation of red blood became possible for the first time. The descent of man is therefore connected with the growth of the tree of the red blood within man.

Just imagine that someone was standing in front of you and you were only aware of the trickling of the red blood; you would have before you a living red tree. Of this Christian esotericism says: It is the Tree of Knowledge. Man has seized it for himself; he has eaten from the tree of red blood. The creation of the Tree of red blood, which is properly the Tree of Knowledge: that is sin. And God drove man out of Paradise, so that he should not also eat of the Tree of Life. We have another tree within us, which you can visualize just as easily as the former. But the latter has blue-red blood. This blood is a poisonous substance. The blue-red tree was planted in man at the same time as the other one. When man still rested in the lap of the Gods, the Godhead within him was capable of interweaving that which signified life and that which signified knowledge—and in future times it will be possible for man, through his

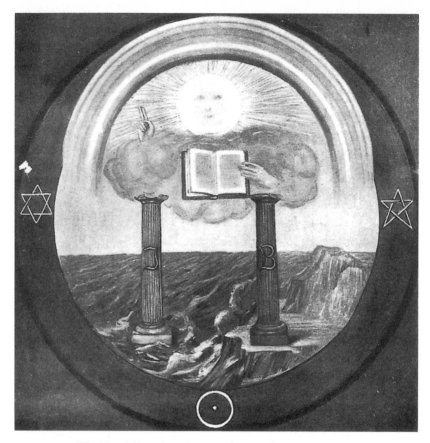

'The Two Pillars' from the 'apocalyptic seals' by Clara Rettich

expanded consciousness, to change the blue-red blood into red blood, then the well-spring will be within himself to change the tree of blue-red blood into a tree of life. Today it is a tree of death. In this picture lies a retrospective and a prophetic view of life!

You see that a tree of red blood and a tree of blue-red blood are intertwined in man. The red blood is the expression of the ego; it is the lower part of ego-knowledge. The blue-red blood gives a picture of death. As a punishment the blue-red tree, as the tree of death, was added to the red tree of knowledge. In the distant future this tree of death will be transformed into the tree of life as it was originally. If you visualize man as he stands before you today, you will see that his whole life consists of interchange between these two trees.[180]

The fact that Seth was allowed to re-enter Paradise signifies that he was an initiate and could look back on the divine-spiritual condition in which the two trees were intertwined. And he laid three seeds of the intertwined trees into Adam's mouth, from which a three-forked tree grew up. That means that the tree which grows out of man, Manas, Budhi and Atman, which comprises his higher members, is present in embryonic form within him. So the legend indicates how already in man's predisposition that is in Adam, the divine Trinity exists—how it grows and develops and how, to begin with, it can only be seen by an initiate. Man has to follow his path of evolution. Everything that has taken place in human development and which leads to initiation is further elaborated in the legend.

Through the knowledge that the tripartite tree resides within us, the tree of eternity which is expressed in the words, 'I am He who was—I am He who is—I am He who will be!' we receive strength which carries us forwards and puts the magical wand into our hand. That is the meaning of Moses' rod; that is why the wood of the tree which grew from the three seeds is taken to the Temple; that is why the Cross is made from it, that sign of initiation which signifies the overcoming of the lower members of man's being by the three higher ones.

This legend thus demonstrates how the initiate looks ahead to a future condition, in which the Tree of Knowledge—the tree of red blood—and the Tree of Life—the tree of blue-red blood—will twine around one another within man himself. Now the one who wishes to advance spiritually should engrave upon his heart what the two pillars—the red pillar on the one hand, indicating the pillar of the red blood, and the blue-red pillar indicating the pillar of the blue-red blood—wish to say to us. Today they are separated from each other. Therefore the red pillar stands on the left in our hall today and the blue-red pillar stands on the right. They are there to indicate to us that we should transcend the present state of mankind and direct our steps to that point in which, through our extended consciousness, the pillars can intertwine in a way which one designates: J B.

'J' denotes the red pillar and 'B' the blue-red one. The inscriptions on the pillars will bring to your mind what is connected with each of them. The words on the red pillar are as follows:

In pure thought you will find	Im reinen Gedanken findest du
The self, which can maintain itself.	Das Selbst, das sich halten kann.
If you transform the thoughts into a picture	Wandelst zum Bilde du den Gedanken,
You will experience creative wisdom.	Erlebst du die schaffende Weisheit.

Whoever mediates this saying engrafts through the power of his thought the column of his red blood with the power that leads him to the goal, to the column of wisdom.

One engrafts the column of life with the power it needs when one gives oneself up to the thought that is inscribed on the other, the blue pillar:

If you condense feeling to become light,	Verdichtest du das Gefühl zum Licht,
You reveal formative power.	Offenbarst du die formende Kraft.
If you embody the will to become entity,	Verdinglichst du den Willen zum Wesen,
You create in universal existence.	So schaffst du im Weltensein.

The one set of words concerns cognition, the other set refers to life. The formative, shaping power reveals itself to begin with in the sense of the first saying; it only becomes 'magical' in the sense of the second saying. To rise from the mere power of cognition to a magical effect lies in the transition from the power of the inscription on the first pillar to that of the inscription on the second.

So you see how what these symbols, the two pillars, denote is linked with the ideals of the Rosicrucian pupil. In some esoteric societies these two pillars are erected. The esotericism will always attach the meaning to them, which has properly been accorded them.[181]

2. An Aspect of the Significance of the Two Pillars. From the Lecture of 20 June 1916 in Berlin. (GA 169)*

It is really true that our passage through life can be compared to the sun moving through the twelve constellations of the zodiac. On entering life our senses rise, as it were, at the one universal pillar and set at the other. We pass by these pillars when we go from the night aspect of the starry heavens into the day aspect. It was to that which these occult or symbolic societies wished to point when they called the pillar of birth—which one passes when one enters the life of the daytime—Jachin. Ultimately they were obliged to seek this pillar in the heavens. And those things which compose our outer existence during our life between death and a new birth are the perceptions we receive from the sense of touch extended over the whole world, in which we do not ourselves do the touching but in which we feel as if we were being touched from all sides by spiritual beings. Here on earth it is we who do the touching. During the life between death and a new birth we live within the movement in such a way that we feel as though within us here a blood corpuscle or a muscle were to sense its own movement. In the macrocosm we feel that we are moving between death and a new birth; we experience ourselves in balance and feel as though we were a part of the whole of life. Here [on earth] our life is enclosed within our skin, there, however, we experience ourselves as a part of the whole of life and in every situation as if we were holding ourselves in balance. Here [on earth] it is the force of gravity and the constitution of our body which gives us our equilibrium, and we actually have no consciousness of it as a rule. We are aware at all times of our equilibrium in the life between death and a new birth. That is an immediate perception, the counterpart to the life of soul. Through Jachin man enters into earthly life and through Jachin one is reassured: 'What is outside of you in the macrocosm now lives within you, you are now a microcosm, for that is the meaning of "Jachin"—the divine in you which is spread out over the world.'

Boaz, the other pillar: Entry through death into the spiritual world. That which is summed up in the word Boaz signifies something like the following: 'I shall find the strength, which I formerly sought within myself, spread out over the whole of existence. I shall live within it.' But one can only understand such things by immersing oneself in them with spiritual insight. In symbolical brotherhoods they are indicated symboli-

---

* Current English edition: *Towards Imagination* (Anthroposophic Press, 1990).

cally. There will be further revelations to come during our fifth post-Atlantean epoch, so that it should not be entirely lost to humanity and so that in later times people can come along who will be able to understand again what has been preserved in the word.

But you see, everything that happens outwardly in our world is, after all, only a picture of what exists outside in the macrocosm. Just as our soul life is a microcosm in the sense I have indicated to you, so is the soul life of all humanity, as it were, formed from without by the macrocosm. And for our present age it is very important to have these two portrayals of the two pillars, of which I have spoken to you, preserved in our history. These pillars give a one-sided picture of life, for life only exists in the equilibrium between the two. Life is not represented either by Jachin, which is only the transition from the spiritual into the bodily, or by Boaz, which is the transition from the bodily into the spirit. The balance is what matters. And that is what mankind finds so difficult to understand. Man is always looking for the one side, for the extreme. He never seeks the balance. That is why two pillars have been erected for our present epoch, but if we interpret our present age correctly, we should pass between the two pillars, imagining neither the one nor the other pillar to be, as it were, the power-base of man's existence. One must pass in between the two! We must really grasp what is present in reality, not brood in thoughtless existence in the way modern materialism broods ...

3. Rudolf Steiner, The Temple Legend,* Extract from Lecture 9 (Third Lecture, Berlin 16 December 1904): The Essence and Task of Freemasonry from the Point of View of Spiritual Science

It is important that we should speak about the higher degrees of Freemasonry ... We are dealing, in the main, with a special rite that is called the combined rite of Memphis and Misraim ...

Now I must mention the various branches of Freemasonry and their tendencies, even if I am only to indicate something briefly. First of all, it is to be borne in mind that the whole of the Masonic higher degrees trace back to a personality often spoken about but equally very much misunderstood. The nineteenth-century historians particularly misunder-

---

* (Rudolf Steiner Press, 1997.)

stood him; they had no idea of the difficult situations an occultist can meet in life. This personality is the ill-famed and little understood Cagliostro. The so-called Count Cagliostro, in whom an individuality concealed itself which was recognized in its true nature only by the highest initiates, attempted originally to bring Freemasonry in London to a higher stage. For during the last third of the eighteenth century Freemasonry had fairly well reached the state that I have described. He did not succeed in London at that time. He then tried in Russia, and also at The Hague. Everywhere he was unsuccessful, for very definite reasons.

Then, however, he was successful in Lyons, forming an occult Masonic Lodge of the Philalethes [Searchers after Truth] out of a group of local Masons, which was called the Lodge of Triumphing Wisdom. Cagliostro specified the purpose of this Lodge. What you can read about it is, however, nothing but the work of ignorant people. What can be said about it is only an indication. Cagliostro was concerned with two things: firstly, with instructions enabling one to produce the so-called Philosopher's Stone; secondly, with creating an understanding of the mystic pentagram. I can only give you a hint of the meaning of these two things. They may be treated with a deal of scorn, but they are not to be taken merely symbolically—they are based on facts.

The Philosopher's Stone has a specific purpose, which is stated by Cagliostro; it is meant to prolong human life to a span of 5,527 years. To a freethinker, that appears laughable. In fact, however, it is possible, by means of special training, to prolong life indefinitely by learning to live outside the physical body. Anyone, however, who imagined that no death, in the conventional sense of the word, could strike down an adept would have quite a false view of the matter. So, whoever imagined that an adept could not be hit and killed by a falling roof slate, would also be wrong. To be sure, that would usually only occur if the adept allowed it. We are not dealing here with physical death, but with the following. Physical death is only an apparent occurrence for him who has understood the Philosopher's Stone for himself, and has learned to separate it. For other people it is a real happening, which signifies a great division in their life. For he who understands how to use the Philosopher's Stone in the way that Cagliostro intended his pupils to do, death is only an apparent occurrence. It does not even constitute a decisive turning-point in life; it is in fact something which is only there for the others who can observe the adept and say that he is dying. He himself, however, does not really die. It is much more the case that the person concerned has learned to live without his physical body, and that he has learned during the course of life to let all those things take place in him gradually which happen suddenly in the physical body at the moment of death. Everything has already taken place in the body of the person concerned which otherwise takes place at death. Death is then no longer possible, for the said person has long ago learned to live without the physical body. He lays aside the physical body in the same way that one takes off a raincoat, and he puts a new body on just as one puts a new raincoat on.

Now that will give you an inkling. That is one lesson which Cagliostro taught—the Philosopher's Stone—which allows physical death to become a matter of small importance.

In the school founded by the Landgrave of Hessen, also, there were two main concerns: the Philosopher's Stone and the knowledge of the pentagram. The Freemasonry founded by the Landgrave of Hessen at that time continued to exist in a rather diluted form. In fact, the whole of Freemasonry, as I have described it, is called the Egyptian rite of Memphis and Misraim. The latter traces its origin back to King Misraim who came from Assyria—from the Orient—and, after the conquest of Egypt, was initiated into the Egyptian mysteries. These are indeed the mysteries which originated from ancient Atlantis. An unbroken tradition exists from that time. Modern Freemasonry is only a continuation of what was established then in Egypt ...

It is correct to say that humanity will be astonished by some of the discoveries that will be made in the near future. But they will be rather premature discoveries and will thereby cause some havoc. The task of the Theosophical Society consists mainly in preparing people for such things. For instance, what I described at the beginning as the knowledge of the Philosopher's Stone was formerly much more universally known than it is today and, indeed, it was known already during a certain period of the Atlantean epoch. At that time the possibility of conquering death was really something which was commonly known ...

The overcoming of death in Atlantean times was naturally preserved in the memories of the individuals concerned without their being aware of it. There are many people reincarnated today who passed through that period in their former lives and who are led to such revelations through their own memories. That will first of all lead to a kind of overrating of certain medical discoveries. People will imagine that medical science was the discoverer of such things. In reality people will have been led to them through their own memories of Atlantean times ...

4. *Rudolf Steiner's Research into the Hiram-St John Individuality, by Hella Wiesberger*★

... If one compiles statements made by Rudolf Steiner on various occasions, it becomes apparent that a decisive factor in this account lies in the importance of the Mystery of Golgotha as the 'conquest over death by the life of the spirit' (Berlin, 23 October 1908). What is to be understood by that follows from the following basic explanation of the relationship between individuality and personality.

> One easily confuses the concepts individuality and personality nowadays. The individuality is that which is eternal and persists from one life to the next. Personality is that which a person brings with him to a single life on earth for its improvement. If we wish to study the individuality we must look at the human soul. If we wish to study the personality we have to look at how the innermost part of man's being expresses itself. The innermost part of man's being is incarnated into a race and into a profession. All of that determines the inner configuration and makes it personal. In the case of a person who is at a lower stage of development, one will notice little of the work upon his inner being. The mode of expression, the kind of gestures and so on conform to those of his race. Those, however, who produce their mode of expression and gestures out of their inner being are more advanced. The more the inner being of a person is able to work on his exterior the more developed he becomes. One could say that the individuality thereby comes to expression within the personality. He who has his own gestures, his own physiognomy, and even has an original character in his way of doing things and in his environment possesses a decided personality. Is that all lost for posterity at death? No, it is not. Christianity knows quite exactly that this is not the case. What is understood by the resurrection of the flesh or the personality is nothing other than the preservation of what is personal throughout all following incarnations. What man has won as a personality remains in his possession, because it is incorporated into his individuality and is carried forward by it into the following incarnations. If we have made something of our body, which is of original character, so will this body and the force that has worked upon it be resurrected. Just so much as we have worked

★ Translated by John Wood.

upon ourselves, and what we have made of ourselves, is preserved. [Berlin, 15 March 1906.]

The real consciousness of immortality is connected therefore with the personalization of the individuality, the higher spiritual members of man's being. And the fact that this process signifies at the same time the Christianization of man is pointed to in the following short commentary to a passage out of the so-called Egyptian Gospel:

> There is an ancient writing in which the highest ideal for the development of the ego, Jesus Christ, is characterized by saying: When the two become one, when the exterior becomes like the interior, then man has attained to Christ-likeness within himself. That is the meaning of a certain passage in the Egyptian Gospel. [Munich, 4 December 1909.]

The meaning of what is within and what is without, of individuality and personality, is made even clearer by the interpretation which Rudolf Steiner gives in his lecture in Berlin on 6 May 1909 to the Provençal saga of Flor and Blancheflor. This saga stands in close connection with the Hiram-John research, because it relates that the soul renowned as Flor reincarnates in the thirteenth and fourteenth centuries as the founder of Rosicrucianism, the mystery school which has as its task the cultivation of the new Christ-secret appropriate to the present day. This saga tells the story of a human pair, born on the same day, at the same hour, in the same house, brought up together and united in love from the very beginning. Separated through the ignorance of others, Flor goes in search of Blancheflor. After difficult and life-threatening dangers they are ultimately reunited until their death, which takes place on the same day as each other.

Rudolf Steiner interprets these scenes in the following way. Flor signifies the flower with the red petals, or the rose, Blancheflor is the flower with the white petals, or the lily. Flor, or the rose, is 'the symbol for the human soul that has taken up into itself the personality or ego-impulse. This allows the spirit to work from its individuality, which has brought the ego-impulse down into the red blood. But in the lily one perceives the symbol of the soul that can only remain spiritual in so far as the ego remains outside it and only approaches as far as the border. Thus rose and lily are two opposites. Rose has self-awareness completely within it, lily has it outside itself. But the merging of the soul that is within and the soul that works from without and enlivens the world as the World Spirit was present. The story of Flor and Blancheflor expresses the discovery of the World Soul, the World Ego, by the human soul, the human ego. (. . .) In the uniting of the Lily-soul and the Rose-soul was envisaged that which can unite with the Mystery of Golgotha.' (Berlin, 6 May 1909.)

When it is said that the uniting of the soul which is within and the soul which enlivens the world from without as the World Spirit 'was present', it is surely the uniting of the Christ principle as the highest spiritual principle with the personality, the earthly body of Jesus of Nazareth, which is referred to. For only through the fact that these two have fully united right down to the physical realm could earthly death truly be conquered.

In how far the contrast of the Rose-soul and Lily-soul can be applied to the two John individualities is shown by the fact that Hiram-Lazarus is always characterized as the representative of the forces of personality, whereas the Elijah-soul is often described as such a highly spiritual being that he can only be loosely connected with his earthly vessels, as was also the case with John the Baptist.[182] If the uniting of the Rose-soul and Lily-soul can lead to union with the Mystery of Golgotha, so may we conclude—in view of the merging of the two John souls at the raising of Lazarus by Jesus Christ—that the disciple whom the Lord loved has become the being to whom the Christ secret of the overcoming of death has become attached and to whom it is still attached, as is expressed in the words which refer to Christian Rosencreutz: 'With this individuality and its activity since the thirteenth century'—by having experienced a further initiation—'we connect all which includes for us the continuation of the impulse given by the appearance of Jesus Christ on earth and through the accomplishment of the Mystery of Golgotha.' (Berlin, 22 December 1912.)

A further aspect follows from this if we combine the words from the Egyptian Gospel 'When the two become one and the exterior becomes the interior' with the second half of the saying, 'and the male becomes like the female, so that there is neither masculine nor feminine'. This latter word points to the fact that there will be no more death when sexuality ceases, for death and sexuality are mutually dependent on one another. Hiram Abiff was already promised in the Temple Legend that a son would be born to him, who, even though he would not see him himself, would give rise to a new race of men. This race, according to Rudolf Steiner, would not know death, because propagation would come about by means of speech and the word connected with the heart and not by means of death-bringing sexuality (Berlin, 23 October 1905). Thus, according to the lecture in Cologne on 2 December 1905, the perfecting of the human race will come about through the raising of the forces of propagation from the womb to the heart, and the 'soul-power of John' will be the force which will raise 'streams of spiritual love' to ray forth from the loving heart. This is hinted at in the Gospel when it describes the scene at the Last Supper in which the disciple whom the Lord loved, who knew the secret of evolution, raised himself from the lap of Christ to His breast.

Against this background all the documents which recount the initiation experiences of the Hiram-Lazarus-John individuality in various incarnations (*The Temple Legend*, *The Gospel of St John*, the Saga of Flor and Blancheflor, *The Chymical Wedding of Christian Rosencreutz anno 1459*, and also the cosmic deed of Christian Rosencreutz at the beginning of the seventeenth century)—by which it was to have been made possible to overcome the polarity of Cain and Abel, both in the single human being as well as in mankind in general—point to the central Christian secret of the conquest of death ...

REFERENCES AND QUOTES

1 Rudolf Steiner, *Occult Science: An Outline*, Rudolf Steiner Press, London, 1963, Chapter IV, 'Man and the evolution of world'.
2 GA 317, lecture 1, Dornach, 25.7.1924
   GA 318, lecture 4, Dornach 13.9.1924
3 *Menschenpersönlichkeitsköper* in German
4 GA 317, lecture 1, Dornach 25.6.24
5 GA 318, lecture 4, Dornach 11.9.24
6 GA 230, lecture 12, Dornach 11.11.1923
7 GA 218, lecture 1, Dornach 20.10.22
8 GA 227, lecture 11, Penmaenmawr 29.8.23
9 GA 99, lecture 5, Munich 29.5.1907
10 GA 235, Volume 1, lecture 5, Dornach 1.3.24
11 GA 318, lecture 4, Dornach 11.9.1924
12 GA 317, lectures 1 and 2, Dornach 2.7.1924, 3.7.1924
13 GA 232, lecture 1, Dornach 23.11.24
14 GA 58, Part I, lecture 5, Munich 14.3.1909
15 GA 145, lecture 10, The Hague 29.3.1913
16 GA 112, lecture 7, Kassel 30.6.1909
17 GA 202, lecture 12, Dornach 19.12.1920
18 Rudolf Steiner, *Knowledge of the Higher Worlds—How is it Achieved?*, Rudolf Steiner Press 1993
19 GA 230, lecture 10, Dornach 9.11.23
20 GA 107, lectures 1 and 2, Berlin 19.10.1908, 21.10.1908
21 GA 128, lecture 3, Prague 22.2.1911
22 Ibid., lectures 6 and 7, Prague 26.3.11, 27.3.1911
23 GA 104, lecture 2, Nuremberg 18.6.1908
   GA 132, lecture 2, Berlin 7.11.1911
24 GA 317, lecture 5, Dornach 30.6.1924
25 GA 230, lecture 11, Dornach 10.11.1923
26 GA 136, lectures 8 and 10, Helsinki 11.4.1912, 13.4.1912
   GA 99, lecture 2, Munich 25.5.1907
27 GA 230, lecture 12, Dornach 11.11.1923
28 GA 93, lecture 15, Berlin 21.10.1905
29 GA 93, lecture 13, Berlin 29.5.1905
30 GA 93, lecture 13, Berlin 29.5.1905
31 GA 131, lecture 10, Karlsruhe 13.10.1911
32 GA 106, lectures 5 and 6, Leipzig 7.11.1908, 8.11.1908
33 GA 95, lecture 10, Stuttgart 31.8.1906

[34] GA 131, lecture 10, Karlsruhe 13.10.1911

[35] GA 93, lecture 9, Berlin 16.12.1904

[36] GA 99, lecture 14, Munich 6.6.1907

[37] GA 245, esoteric lesson, Berlin 2.10.1906

[38] GA 93, lecture 3, Berlin 16.12.1904

[39] GA 318, lecture 11, Dornach 18.9.1924

[40] GA 318, lecture 11, Dornach 18.9.1924

[41] *Fundamentals of Therapy*, Chapter XVII. (See also Appendix to Chapter 2. Current edition: *Extending Practical Medicine*, Rudolf Steiner Press, London 1996.)

[42] GA 232, lecture 14, Dornach 23.12.1923

[43] GA 317, lecture 5, Dornach 30.6.1924

[44] GA 202, lecture 12, Dornach 19.12.1920

[45] GA 318, lectures 7 and 8, Dornach 15.9.1924

[46] GA 319, lecture 6, The Hague 16.11.23

Calcium–phosphor polarity: Phosphor is the driving motor of inhalation, of all breathing processes inwardly directed. It conveys air into the human organization in a way that gives it a warming influence on the nerve-sense organization. But because calcium carbonate has a dispelling, excreting effect, it clears the way in the human organism for the astral body and ego organization to function. It is because of what calcium carbonate drives out that the astral body and ego organization can enter man, whereas what phosphor drives into the physical organization forces the astral body and ego out. This is why phosphor facilitates sleep.

[47] Degenaar, page 110: Doctors' discussion on influenza, 23.5.1922

Phosphor and calcium (reported by Dr Husemann 1922)

Phosphor is a latent combustion process. Does it bring about a greater liquidity of the blood? No, it calls forth these inner oxidation processes and keeps them aflame in the organism; it prevents the blood from emerging from a febrile condition. Its liquidity effect is secondary . . .

[48] GA 319, lecture 1, Penmaenmawr 28.8.1923

Phosphor regulates those forces that are really a kind of organic combustion process—which is always present when substances are transformed in the human organism.

Each time we move, or whenever we eat, organic combustion processes occur . . . If the organism has become too weak to limit organic combustion processes in the right way, then . . . tuberculosis arises . . . The right conditions are created for the bacilli when a capacity to limit combustion processes is lacking . . . If one now treats the organism with phosphor, one supports these capacities of limiting organic combustion processes, of keeping them in proper bounds.

Degenaar appendix, doctors' conference IV, 1922

Doctors' discussion IV, 1922: 'Fever'

Simply imagine that you are in a terribly expectant mood. In relation to the sense system this means that you urgently wish your sense impressions to follow one another in quick succession. So initially you fall into a soul fever. Continue this process in your imagination and you get the effect of phosphor. The inflammatory process arises, after all, from the fact that there is too strong a phosphor activity in the organism. The will process consists in the combustion of organic substance. If you have too strong an inner inflammatory process, you will develop an inward condition equivalent to outer sense impressions following one another in the most rapid succession. If your normal temperature were a great deal higher, the world would have to be experienced far more swiftly . . .
GA 347, lecture 6, Dornach 16.9.1922
It is actually the case that a kind of phosphor arises from the food we eat, so that food does not simply penetrate up into the head. Much forces its way upwards: sugar, glycerine etc., all sorts of things do, but part of it is transformed into phosphor before it rises upwards . . . Thus we have salts in our head which have been taken up almost unchanged from the outer world. Similarly, in a gaseous, finely distributed form—actually much more rarefied than air, we have phosphor distributed in us. These are the chief substances in the human head, salts and phosphor . . . one needs a good quantity of salt in one's head to be able to think properly . . . It is because we have phosphor that the will is there. And when we have too much phosphor, this will begins to flail about . . . the human being starts . . . flailing around nervously, agitatedly . . . gets into a frenzy.

[49] *Fundamentals of Therapy*, Chapter XII
Phosphor is effective as a remedy if the astral organization predominates over the ego organization and where the latter needs strengthening to hold sway over the astral organization.

[50] GA 313, lecture 5, Dornach 15.4.1921
. . . the human ego is . . . from a spiritual, emotional, organic and also mineralizing point of view . . . a kind . . . of phosphor-bearer . . . This phosphor-bearing is carried out by the ego in an extraordinarily adept way, right to the furthest boundaries, right to the periphery of the organic human organism . . . [and it] belongs to the ego's task, in bearing phosphor through the organism . . . to prevent its chemical release, except for the phosphor traces that are needed . . . As the ego works to establish equilibrium from unbalanced conditions, it needs phosphor . . . What the ego does must reach all the way to the blood corpuscles.' . . . Concealed battle between the continual phosphorizing of man and what lies in the structuring blood process . . . 'If phosphor is carried in a free state into the human organism, then the blood corpuscles are destroyed by the phosphorizing process . . .

[51] GA 314, lecture 4, Dornach 9.10.1920

By treating someone with too strong a phosphor dose, in a certain sense one can separate out what is the bearer of the ego activity in the physical body from this ego activity itself, so that this ego activity is carried out in the body alone as though in a (physical) reflection. This would lead to a kind of hyperaemia, excess blood activity, which would work against the calcification process of the bones. And we must gain insight into the fact that when rickets arises in the human organism this is a similar process to what happens when phosphor arises outside in nature ... In the human head system [we] always [have] certain functions that derive from phosphor, which are found in man's brain. In the brain we have a continual ... kind of emerging rickets. This is the very thing that our brain activity depends on—that there is a continual tendency towards a bone-formation process, but that this is continually prevented once the skull bone has been properly formed around the brain ... and in a broader sense phosphor is a general remedy that counteracts every pathological emancipation of ego activity within the physical body from actual soul activity, and reunites it with soul activity, i.e. returns it to a normal condition.
GA 351, lecture 5, Dornach 5.12.23
... One should treat arteriosclerosis of the brain with Phosphor preparations ...

[52] GA 319, lecture 6, The Hague 16.11.1923
If we observe this process in the sense organs, which turns out to be identical with the quartz process, we come to see—and mineralogy shows us the same thing in outer nature—that the quartz process is least able to work harmoniously with the phosphor process ... and by means of this interaction between a process such as the phosphor process and another such as the silica process the eye becomes an organ whose physical organization the ego and astral body present in man can take hold of.

[53] GA 313, lecture 2, Dornach 12.4.1921
... the effect of small traces of phosphor and sulphur is that they expel the astral body that has penetrated the physical and etheric bodies too deeply. Sulphur does this more to the astral body and phosphor more to the ego, which, however of course, since it permeates and organizes the astral body, really works with it as a unity ... When the ego and astral body take too strong a hold of the head and respiratory organization, attack them too strongly ... it is difficult to fall asleep. [Author's note: Phosphor and sulphur help to expel the astral body and ego organization.]
Fundamentals of Therapy, Chapter XV
Strong etheric oils, particularly from plant blossoms, also phosphor-containing substances, can relieve the astral body and ego organization of the activity that is not rightfully theirs.

[54] Ala Selawry, Metallfuktionstypen in Psychologie und Medizin, Haug Verlag, Stuttgart. 'Zinn-Kapitel'

55 Ala Selawry, *Metallfuktionstypen in Psychologie und Medizin*, Haug Verlag, Stuttgart. 'Blei-, Zinn-und Eisen-Kapitel'

56 *Fundamentals of Therapy*, Chapter XV
Phosphor sustains the ego organization, so that it can overcome the physical body's opposition.

57 GA 319, lecture 6, The Hague 16.11.1923
Calcium carbonate has the tendency in the human organism to exert an excretory effect ... calcium reveals man's centrifugal, outward radiating forces in outer nature ... if these outward radiating forces become too strong, thus giving rise to illness, one can diminish these processes of illness ... through calcium preparations ... The calcium forces localized in the human being are also all that underlies human exhalation. Calcium has within it the strength which acts as the motor of exhalation ... Thus in our lower sphere, in the metabolic-limb system, it has an excretory effect on fluids, in our rhythmic sphere it dispels gaseous substances, and in the nerve-sense organization it drives out the warmth ether ... In each of these connections calcium has an opposite effect to phosphor [see Phosphorus]. It is precisely through what calcium drives out that the astral body and ego organization can enter man ... The calcium function, when the phosphor function does not counteract it, is a continual cause of us entering into all those processes connected with insomnia.

58 GA 348, lecture 16, Dornach 27.1.1923
Respiratory process: But carbon dioxide arises as a result. Yes, this carbon dioxide, it is mostly expelled. But if all carbon dioxide left our bodies, we humans would all be as thick as two planks—for part of the carbon dioxide must continually pass into our nervous system ... The nervous system needs this deadening carbon dioxide. So part of the carbon dioxide simply rises in me as interior air, and supplies my nervous system ... The breath-poison of carbon dioxide continually streams up into my head, and it is this breath-poison that enables me to think.
GA 208, lecture 6, Dornach 30.10.21
Man takes up this enlivening oxygen, which is connected with his limb system, with everything in him that moves. He combines the oxygen with carbon. The carbon initially has a stimulating effect, which devitalizes our nerve-sense life, then it is expelled as something dying. Thus we have, in material terms, the most extreme life in oxygen, and the most extreme death in carbon ...

59 *Fundamentals of Therapy*, Chapter VI
The portion of carbon dioxide that passes into the head with metabolism there assumes the tendency, through combining with calcium, to enter into the workings of the ego organization. As a result calcium carbonate is driven towards bone-formation under the influence of the head-nerves, which are inwardly stimulated by the ego organization.

[60] GA 327, lecture 3, Koberwitz 11.6.1924

In order for what lives in carbon to be flexible, able to move, man creates in his calcium carbonate-based skeletal framework an underlying solidity ... In so doing man elevates himself, with his mobile carbon structure, from merely mineral, solid calcium carbonate such as the earth has, and which he integrates into himself so that he can contain solid earth. Calcium gives carbon earthly formative forces, while silica gives it cosmic formative force ... But we also find calcium and silica as the basis of plant growth ...

[61] GA 327, lecture 1, Koberwitz 7.6.1924

Moon, Mercury and Venus, via Calcium carbonicum, work down upon earth's plant and animal life.

[62] *Fundamentals of Therapy*, Chapter XVI

The organism is chiefly formed through transformation of protein substance, by means of which the latter interacts and links with mineralizing forces—as contained in calcium carbonate for example. The way the oyster forms its shell provides an image of this process. The oyster has to rid itself of what goes to make its shell, so as to retain its own protein substance in its own nature. Something similar occurs in eggshell formation ... This integration must take place in the human organism. The protein process as such must be transformed into one in which are involved structuring forces that the ego organization can call forth in calcareous substance.

[63] GA 319, lecture 1, Penmaenmawr 28.8.1923

Calcium remedies using animal calcium excretions ... bring about the right relationship between the body of formative forces and the physical body ...

[64] GA 312, lecture 5, Dornach 25.3.1920

The oyster builds up its calcium carbonate house from within outwards. If you ... research into the oyster from a spiritual-scientific perspective, you will come to recognize that although it is a very low form of animal life, it occupies a relatively elevated position in the whole cosmos ... through the fact that ... it expels what man bears within him as his thinking ... And in the way the oyster shell forms, you have a tangible image of the work of calcium carbonate ... which leads excessive soul-spiritual activity out of the organism. If you find, therefore, that there is excessive soul-spiritual activity in the lower body ... you will need to have recourse to a remedy which we have the oyster shell to thank for.

[65] GA 348, lecture 2, Dornach, 24.10.1922

The brain can also calcify. It must always have a little of what occurs through the calcification process. You see, a child without a little calcium carbonate sand in his head, which the pineal gland excretes and spreads about, would stay stupid, the soul would be unable to enter, for it finds its way in through calcium carbonate. But later, when an old person has too much calcium carbonate in his system, everything hardens and he becomes senile; and then, once again, the soul is unable to get a proper grasp [on the brain], for this [hardening] is too strong ... Then one is removed again from earthly forces.

[66] *Fundamentals of Therapy*, Chapter VI

See quote 59.

[67] GA 314, lecture 4, Dornach 9.10.1920

Under the influence of phosphor forces [and sulphur forces—the author], there is a kind of hyperaemia in the bone system. This hyperaemia ... would counter the calcification process of the bones.

[68] Degenaar appendix, Hippocrates-Kalk (1922)

The calcium carbonate content of the brain is higher in a new-born baby than later on ... The calcium carbonate that is here present, in what one can call pieces—in grains—enables pre-embryonic soul-life to participate in forming the brain. This is not the case in animals, where the calcium carbonate goes straight into forming the skull. The child arrives in the world in a less mature state than the anthropoids. Thus the fact that calcium carbonate is retained in the brain signifies de-animalization; and loss of calcium means falling back into animal existence, and increased hypersensitivity. But de-animalization also occurs through other substances ... Old-age sclerosis occurs through calcium entering the organism via the metabolic system. The chief deposit of calcium carbonate is in the pineal gland. When it is lacking there, the child suffers from idiocy ... During the course of life, they [the calcium carbonate grains] continually dissolve and re-form ... In the infant calcium carbonate exerts a material effect; later this becomes functional when the human being takes over the role of calcium carbonate.

GA 348, lecture 2, Dornach 24.10.1922

See quote 65.

[69] GA 312, lecture 6, Dornach 26.3.1920

This is why doctors who have a certain success in treating rickets with phosphor will probably not have the slightest success in treating craniotabes. Here a quite opposite treatment is needed, using a remedy with some kind of calcium carbonate or suchlike.

[70] GA 319, lecture 6, The Hague 16.11.1923

See quote 57.

[71] Degenaar appendix, Phosphor und Kalzium (1922)

Phosphor and calcium: With calcium carbonate are connected all the conditions of anxiety and fear. Under its influence a person would become all head, would grow pale ... If calcium alone exerted its influence on man, it would cause us to become all head. One should give calcium carbonate in anaemic and consumptive conditions, but in a highly diluted form—if one administers it directly, it easily puts down deposits in the organism ...

[72] GA 349, lecture 2, Dornach 21.2.1923

So in a pale child like this, all the carbon within him is continually transformed into carbon dioxide. This is what makes him pale. So what must I do? I must administer something which hinders this continual forming of carbon dioxide inside him, which enables the carbon to be retained. I can do this by giving him some calcium carbonate. By so doing, as I explained to you from a quite different perspective, the child's bodily functions are stimulated once more, and he retains the carbon, which he needs, no longer transforming it continually into carbon dioxide.

[73] Degenaar appendix, Hippocrates-Kalk (1922)
See quote 68.

[74] GA 319, lecture 6, The Hague 16.11.23
In outer nature, where we find silica, quartz ... we have something which corresponds to what unfolds in the human organism, in the eye for instance or another sense organ. One cannot say that there is actually quartz substance there, but what we have in the eye or other sense organs is, in functional terms, the same process that quartz manifests in nature.
GA 239, lecture 15, Breslau 14.6.24
The way that they [the sense organs] are at present, reflecting the outer world within, only evolved at a relatively late stage—at the same time, for example, as silica in its present form evolved on earth ... This is why silica, when properly used as a remedy, affects everything throughout the human body that is related to the nerve-sense system, to the senses. The senses in their present state were formed last of all, at the same time that the rocks in which silica in its present state is contained were also formed.

[75] GA 347, lecture 3, Dornach 9.8.22
Just as carbon dioxide arises in us when we exhale, so, when silica in the earth properly combines with oxygen, quartz silicic acid arises ... But oxygen does not in itself have the capacity to combine with silicium ... Why do these beautiful forms come about? Yes, they form by themselves, because forces stream in from all sides of the cosmos, and the earth is in continual relationship and connection with the whole cosmos ... Thus all these crystals arise from the fact that the earth is influenced by all the other planets and stars. So we can say that these crystals are really formed by the cosmos ... in the cosmos everything is ordered in a crystalline way ... In our nerves there are miniscule silica crystals, which must continually dissolve. When such very tiny crystals collect in the nervous system, we get tiny pinpricks that people do not know how to explain ... Small inflammations also come about ... and then a person gets rheumatism or gout ... If we have no brain-sand we become stupid. If these crystals formed [in the brain], we would continually faint, for, one can say, we would get brain-rheumatism, or brain-gout. In the rest of the body it only causes pain; but when the brain contains these minuscule crystals, one is incapacitated and faints ... To look at something [very attentively] is really the same as a tiny flower forming from the brain-sand in us, except that the flower grows from above downwards ... Just think, a flower, for instance, tries to form within us a lifeless silica image of

itself. That mustn't happen, for otherwise we would know nothing about the flower, but just get 'head-gout'. It first has to dissolve ... This dissolving means that man can think of himself in such a way as to be able to say 'I'. Saying 'I' makes the brain-sand dissolve most of all.

[76] GA 319, lecture 11, London 29.8.24

Thus we can say that the spirit of such a rock crystal has, for instance, a particularly strong effect on man's ego organization. Man's ego organization, when it bears the essence of silica within it for example, gains mastery of the spirit of silica, in other words of quartz. That is the significant thing.

[77] GA 351, lecture 10, Dornach 1.12.23

If you go into high mountainous regions you will find quartz crystals precisely where the mountain rock is hardest, where, one can say, the hardest earth substance is built ... The earth lets hexagonal, pointed crystals grow out of itself. In the earth, therefore, lies the force to create such hexagonal forms ... This force, which impels quartz crystals out of the earth, is also within man. How does it manifest? Yes, the human body is full of quartz ... So hardness is the striking thing about quartz. But substances do not manifest everywhere in the same form. Inside the human being there is the very same substance as quartz, but in a more fluid form. Why? That is very interesting. If you look at the human head, the same thing is continually streaming down from the head as once streamed from within the earth outwards, which then grew hard and deposited itself as quartz crystals for instance ... But the human body does not allow the quartz to become crystalline ... The human organism lets it get to the point where it would just be about to become hexagonal ... so that in our bodies we only have the first beginnings of crystalline formation ... And our life depends on the fact that we are continually trying to form hexagonal crystals from above downwards, but not let it get as far as that, stop before it does ... and inside us we have, as it were, quartz juice in highly diluted form. If we didn't have this quartz juice, for instance, however much sugar we ate we would never have a sweet taste in our mouths. This is what the quartz does which we have within us, but not through its material substance; rather through the fact that it has the will, is striving, to become a hexagonal crystal ... But one can do something else. One can give people highly diluted, powdered quartz—silica—as a remedy—then they will become able, after a while, to benefit from small quantities of honey. This highly diluted silica has then awakened the strength within them to activate hexagonal, crystallizing forces, and then a small quantity of honey can follow. Thus the silica can prepare the way for the honey.

[78] GA 319, lecture 1, Penmaenmawr 28.8.1923

So if one introduces this silica-forming process into the human organism, it supports an underactive nerve-sense system ... Thus one can see in the forces active in silica ... that they are particularly suited for re-establishing the right relationship between the ego and the astral body, and thus for exerting a healing effect on the nerve-sense system ... and those processes which correspond to the silica process are found in the root organs of plants.

[79] GA 319, lecture 9, Arnheim 24.7.24

Discussion of migraine: How do we reintroduce the ego organization into the actual nervous system, into this continuation of the nerves from outside inwards? How do we drive the ego back to the place it has withdrawn from, the central portions of the brain? We do this ... by administering silica. But if we only used silica, we would make the ego integrate into the central nerve-sense organization of the head, it is true, but would still leave the surrounding areas—the grey matter of the brain—as it is ...

[80] *Fundamentals of Therapy*, Chapter XV

Where there are inflammatory symptoms of the skin, the astral body and the ego organization develop abnormal activity ... If one administers silica to the organism, the activities of the astral and the ego organization are relieved from focusing on the skin. The inwardly-directed activity of these organisms is released once more, and a healing process begins.

[81] GA 319, lecture 1, Penmaenmawr 28.8.1923

See quote 78.

[82] *Fundamentals of Therapy*, Chapter XIX

In therapy we are concerned to diminish the sensitivity of the astral body and ego organization. We can do this by administering silica, which always strengthens the organism's inner forces against over-sensitivity. In this case we did this by adding powdered silica to food, and administering it as an enema.

[83] GA 354, lecture 2, Dornach 3.7.1924

Silica is a very precious remedy. When one realizes that the human digestion works properly, but that this digestion process cannot reach the sense organs, the head or the skin, one should use silica as a remedy.

[84] *Fundamentals of Therapy*, Chapter XIV

Silica carries its effects, via metabolism, into the parts of the human organism in which living substances become lifeless. It appears in the blood, through which the formative forces must pass; and it appears in the hair—in other words where the structure [of the organism] closes itself to the outside world; also in the bones, where structuring forces come to an end inside us. It appears in the urine as a product of excretion. It forms the physical basis of the ego organization, for the latter has a structuring effect. This ego organization needs the silica process to penetrate right into the parts of the organism in which structure and form border on the outer and inner (unconscious) world ...

The physical basis of consciousness needs to develop between silica's two fields of activity in the healthy human organism. Silica has a twofold task. Within, it sets limits to processes of mere growth and nutrition. And towards the outer world it closes the organism off from merely natural influences, so that it does not have to continue these natural effects within its own realm ... One can really speak of a specific silica organism integrated into the overall organism. On this depends the organs' mutual responses to one another—which underlie healthy life—as well as their proper relationships, within to the soul and spirit, and without to properly closing off the organism from natural influences.

85 GA 327, lectures 1 and 2, Koberwitz 7.6.1924, 10.6.1924
    Lecture 1, 'Silica-calcium Polarity: Cosmic and Terrestrial'
    Lecture 2:
    On the circuitous path via ... siliceous sand, what mainly comes into the soil and then works back through reflection ... is what we can call the earth's etheric life and its chemical activity. To what extent the soil itself becomes inwardly alive, exerts its own chemical activity is very much dependent on the nature of this soil's sandy constituency. And what the plants' roots experience in the soil is again largely dependent on the extent to which cosmic life and cosmic chemical ether have been collected and gathered on this round-about path via the [silica] rock ...
    He [man] does not know that this cosmic stone, silica, is what receives light into the earth, makes it active there ...

86 *Fundamentals of Therapy*, Chapter XIV
    See quote 84.

87 GA 318, lecture 7, Dornach 14.9.24
    See Chapter 4.

88 GA 230, lecture 10, Dornach 9.11.1923
    If we follow metabolism up into the breathing, we will actually find that man forms out of himself the carbon that is to be found everywhere within him. This carbon is sought by oxygen and transformed into carbon dioxide, which we then exhale ... The oxygen breathed in ... takes up carbon into itself; and we breathe out carbon dioxide. But before exhalation takes place, one can say that carbon performs benevolent services to human nature. In uniting with oxygen, in joining what in a certain sense brings about blood circulation and with what respiration then achieves through this blood circulation ... carbon spreads through the whole human organism an emanation of ether before it departs from us ... This ether penetrates the human etheric body. And this ether, produced by carbon, is the very thing that renders the human organization suitable for opening itself to spiritual influences, it is what takes up astral-etheric influences from the cosmos. This ether left behind by carbon attracts the cosmic impulses which, in turn, work formatively back upon man, and which, for instance, make his nervous system capable of sustaining thoughts. This ether must continually permeate our senses—our eyes for instance, so that they can see, so that they can take up the outer light ether. Thus we owe it to carbon that we

have within us an ether preparation, which can open to and receive the world.

[89] GA 213, lecture 5, Dornach 2.7.22

... if man, as it were, only had quartz-like forces in himself, he would continually be in danger of his soul-spirit striving back towards what he was between death and a new birth, before he sets foot on the earth. Quartz tries continually to lift man out of himself, and return him to his discarnate being. Another force is needed to oppose this one, which tries to return man to his incarnated being; and that is the force of carbon ... But when one understands this fully, one sees on the other hand what healing forces silicium, quartz or silica, contains. If someone falls ill through a too strong carbon process, which is the case in all illnesses connected with certain metabolic products deposited by metabolism, he needs silica as a remedy. Silica is particularly effective where deposits are peripheral or in the head.

[90] GA 347, lecture 3, Dornach 9.8.22

See quote 75.

[91] *Beiträge zur Rudolf Steiner Gesamtausgabe*, Heft 20, Seite 20.

Through remedies that affect the metabolism, the healing power of the will is activated—Sulphur heals through the will.

[92] GA 314, lecture 5, Dornach 9.10.20

If we introduce such a blossom, or even only the sulphur extracted from such a plant, as a remedy into the human organism, then above all we stimulate what occurs in the digestive tract to greater activity ... And when we succeed, by means of external or internal sulphur treatment ... in stimulating the digestive tract so strongly that it stimulates the activity of heart and lungs in turn, so that the kidney activity once more collects and absorbs the material ... then we can certainly manage to overcome metabolic illnesses.

[93] *Fundamentals of Therapy*, Chapter XX

Sulphur 'contains the process whereby the rhythm tending towards the digestive system is transformed into that tending towards breathing'.

[94] GA 327, lecture 3, Koberwitz 11.6.24

On the importance of sulphur in forming protein: For sulphur is the very thing within protein which acts as a mediator between the spirit spread out everywhere in the cosmos, between the formative force of the spirit and the physical. And anyone ... who wishes to follow the traces which the spirit leaves in the material world must follow the activity of sulphur ... And this is why substances such as sulphur and phosphor, which are connected with the influx of light into matter, were called light-bearers ...

... just as the human ego, as the real spirit of the human being, lives in carbon, so one can say the cosmic ego in the cosmic spirit lives, via sulphur, in the forming and dissolving of carbon ... this physical substance that, with the help of sulphur, carries life forces out of the etheric, is oxygen ... on a circuitous path via sulphur ...

95 *Fundamentals of Therapy*, Chapter XIII

Look at sulphur. This is contained in protein ... it thus reveals itself as a substance that plays a role in the absorption of protein substance into the realm of the human etheric body ... It unfolds its activity in the realm of the physical and the etheric body ... Sleep ... becomes deeper through increased doses of sulphur.

From this one can see that, administered as a remedy, sulphur makes the organism's physical activities more open to the influence of the etheric than they are in a state of illness. If one treats [rickets] with sulphur ... the etheric is strengthened in contrast to astral activity ...

96 GA 351, lecture 2, Dornach 10.10.1923

The moon once departed from the earth, endowing the air with oxygen and the soil with carbon.

GA 233, lecture 7, Dornach 20.12.23

We have substances that are subject to earthly nature ... black coal. What is it in reality? This is only black coal in the vicinity of the earth, for if it were taken only a short distance away from the earth, it would no longer be as it is. Coal becomes coal solely by virtue of earth forces.

GA 316, lecture 3, Dornach 4.1.1924

You see, there is diamond, graphite, anthracite and coal—and they are all carbon, yet in such different forms. Why is that? If, besides the mere chemical composition of a substance, people could really sense what used to be thought of as its 'signature', they would begin to understand the difference between coal and graphite. Coal arose during the stage of Earth evolution, while graphite came about during Moon evolution, the planetary stage preceding the earth; and diamond arose during Sun evolution.

97 GA 97, lecture 24, Leipzig 16.2.1907

Fourthly: discovering the Philosopher's Stone ... The Philosopher's Stone is the highest and noblest stage man can attain, to which he can develop his organism so as to reach a higher stage of evolution ... Man has carbon within him; he inhales oxygen and carbon dioxide is produced, which is then disposed of ... Now the Rosicrucians teach a special forming of the breathing process, through which human beings can learn the process that the plant undertakes. Then man will be able to transform carbon within him, he will be able to transform blue arterial blood into red again. He thus takes up the plant's nature into himself, and will one day be able to do what the plant can do now. Man is working towards this ideal of forming his own body from carbon—ordinary coal is the Philosopher's Stone. It will not appear as black coal, but as transparent, clear, bright carbon, once man's body has become starlike. These are not only chemical processes but also high ideals.

[98] GA 284, lecture 1, Munich 19.5.1907

We actually need do nothing other than observe the process that cosmically sustains us in the present epoch: the breathing process. We breathe in and out: inhale the air's oxygen, and give back to the outer world carbon dioxide, a poisonous gas in which we could not live. The plant continually takes this up, retains the carbon and from it builds up its own substance, but gives oxygen back to the animals and human beings. Thus plant, animal and man form an interacting whole, as far as their bodily substance is concerned. Nowadays man needs the plant. The corpse of the plant as black coal, which we dig up, or also transparent diamond, is something which we have within us as well, but we cannot use it ... The plant builds its structure from carbon dioxide itself ... Now just picture this process to yourself: intake of carbon dioxide by the plant, and its emitting of oxygen, and think of this process transferred into the interior of human beings ... thus a merging with the plant world comes about, which is taken up into human nature. Then we will build up in ourselves, as the plant does already, a pure, chaste body ... The breathing process is not completed; what now happens outside us will gradually become transposed into our interior ... Carbon is the substance of which the human body will in future be built.

GA 93a, lecture 4, Berlin 29.9.1905

Man ... takes up oxygen into himself and transforms it through his life processes into carbon dioxide, by combining it with carbon. The plants build up their substance from the carbon, which they retain ... If you look at a piece of coal, you can say that this was once formed from plant life ... exactly the same can be said of a diamond. Nature has formed diamond out of a coal that was still older than the one we observe. Quartz crystal also arose from plants ... Man will then, consciously, go through the same process of working upon carbon that nowadays plants undergo unconsciously. He will transform substance just as the plant nowadays transforms air into carbon. That is true alchemy. Coal is the Philosopher's Stone ... Man's body will in future also be built from carbon, and he will then be something like a soft diamond.

GA 100, lecture 14 Kassel 9.6.07

The relationship between man and the plant world ...

Man continually takes in oxygen, thus sustaining his body, and breathes out carbon dioxide: he himself therefore continually produces a poison, which would kill him ... What does the plant do? ... It takes up this carbon dioxide, retains the carbon from it, and emits the oxygen which is of no use to it ... What does the plant do with the carbon which it retains? The plant uses this to some extent to build up its own substance. In a certain sense, then, we give the plant the opportunity of building itself up out of carbon. When coal is dug up out of the earth after thousands of years, the same substance is still present ... that is a wonderful mutual interaction. This is how it is nowadays ... in future man will bear a body free of desires, of a higher order, which one can already see today at a lower stage in plants. He will be able to build up a body that is plantlike at a higher stage. In other words, what the plant now does outside us will later occur within us, and we will then retain the carbon, which nowadays we dispose of, within ourselves, and use it to build up our own bodies ... The Philosopher's Stone is ordinary black coal, but you need to learn the process which teaches you to work upon this carbon through inner strength: this is man's progressive path. In coal nowadays we have an image and precursor of what will one day be the most important substance for human beings. Remember the bright diamond—that is only carbon!

[99] GA 131, lecture 7, Karlsruhe 10.10.1911

So what renders man visible? The luciferic forces within him make him visible in the way that we encounter him on the physical plane; otherwise his [the human being's] physical body would have remained invisible. This is why the alchemists have always stressed that the human body in reality consists of the same substance that composes the wholly transparent, wax-soft Philosopher's Stone. The physical body is actually composed of absolute transparency, and the luciferic forces in the human being are what have brought it to this state of opacity ...

[100] GA 93, lecture 3, Berlin 29.5.1905

See Appendix to Chapter 2.

[101] GA 284, lecture 1, Munich 19.5.1907

See quote 98.

GA 93a, lecture 4, Berlin 29.9.1905

See quote 98.

[102] See Chapter 3.

[103] See Chapter 6.

[104] GA 314, lecture 2, Dornach 7.4.20

Carbon underpins the animal, plant and human organizations by fixing and determining the physical organization ...

[105] GA 327, lecture 3, Koberwitz 7.6.24

When the old alchemists spoke of the Philosopher's Stone, they were referring to all the various forms of carbon ... And why was it carbon? ... Carbon is the bearer of all structuring processes in nature ... Carbon is the great sculptor which, when fully active and inwardly mobile, bears within itself everywhere formative cosmic pictures, the great cosmic imaginations out of which all that is formed in nature must arise. There is a secret sculptor at work in carbon ... The active spirit of the universe ... works as a sculptor and, with the help of carbon, builds up the more solid plant-form; but then also builds up the form of the human being that dissipates even as it arises— which is in fact human, not plant, by virtue of the fact that we can always immediately destroy the form that has arisen by exhaling carbon bound up with oxygen, as carbon dioxide ... Thus our breathing immediately breaks down what has been formed, tears this carbon out of its solidity, links it with oxygen, conveys it outwards, and in this way we are endowed with the fluidity we need as human beings.

[106] GA 351, lecture 2, Dornach 10.10.1923

Nitrogen ... goes hand-in-hand with carbon in brotherly fashion. Carbon is contained in coal, diamond and in graphite. But carbon is also in us—though there it is fluid and swims about.

[107] GA 319, lecture 6, The Hague 16.11.1923
See quote 46.

[108] GA 93a, lecture 29, Berlin 3.11.1905

In the middle of Lemurian times the respiratory process began to assume the form that it has today ... Breathing is a material image of the spiritual process of the embedding of the monads [ego and Spirit Self, Life Spirit and Spirit Man—the author] in the lower man [astral body, etheric body and physical body—the author]. Breathing means: the monads enter ... Pneuma means 'a breath' and also the soul-spirit ... For the taking up of spirit corresponds with gaseous respiration ...

[109] GA 319, lecture 1, Penmaenmawr 28.8.1923

Phosphor regulates those forces that are really a kind of organic combustion process—which is always present when substances are transformed in the human organism.

Each time we move, or whenever we eat, organic combustion processes occur ...

[110] GA 351, lecture 2, Dornach 10.10.1923
See quote 106.

[111] GA 230, lecture 10, Dornach 9.11.1923

If we follow metabolism up into the breathing, we will actually find that man forms out of himself the carbon that is to be found everywhere within him. This carbon is sought by oxygen and transformed into carbon dioxide, which we then exhale ... The oxygen breathed in ... takes up carbon into itself; and we breathe out carbon dioxide. But before exhalation takes place, one can say that carbon performs benevolent services to human nature. In uniting with oxygen, in joining what in a certain sense brings about blood circulation with what respiration then achieves through this blood circulation ... carbon spreads through the whole human organism an emanation of ether before it departs from us ... This ether penetrates the human etheric body. And this ether, produced by carbon, is the very thing that renders the human organization suitable for opening itself to spiritual influences, is what takes up astral-etheric influences from the cosmos. This ether left behind by carbon attracts the cosmic impulses which, in turn, work formatively back upon man, and which, for instance, make his nervous system capable of sustaining thoughts. This ether must continually permeate our senses—our eyes for instance, so that they can see, so that they can take up the outer light-ether. Thus we owe it to carbon that we have within us an ether preparation which can open to and receive the world.

[112] GA 314, lecture 2, Dornach 7.4.20
See quote 104.

[113] *Beiträge zur Rudolf Steiner Gesamtausgabe*, Heft 35, Seite 13
Carbon dioxide is related to man as he is today; it destroys form—stimulates digestion—serves all that has not yet been worked on by the digestive secretions ... Wherever we notice a lack of what carbon dioxide carries out, we need to administer high potency carbon dioxide.

[114] *Fundamentals of Therapy*, Chapter XX
Sulphur 'contains the process whereby the rhythm tending towards the digestive system is transformed into that tending towards breathing'.

[115] *Fundamentals of Therapy*, Chapter VI
The carbon dioxide involved in exhalation, before it leaves the body, is chiefly composed of merely living—neither sentient nor dead—substance ... The large proportion of this living carbon dioxide leaves the organism, but a small amount remains behind and continues to work into the processes centred in the head organization ... The carbon dioxide expelled from the body through exhalation is living substance as long as it is still in the body; the astral activity anchored in the central nervous system grasps hold of it and expels it.

[116] GA 319, lecture 6, The Hague 16.11.23
The calcium forces localized in the human organism are thus also what underpin human exhalation. Calcium carbonate contains within it the power which drives exhalation ... In the human being's lower sphere, therefore, in the metabolic-limb system, it exerts an excretory effect on fluids; in the rhythmic sphere it works to expel gaseous substance; and in the nerve-sense organization it drives out the warmth ether ...

[117] GA 348, lecture 16, Dornach 27.1.23
Breathing process: But carbon dioxide arises as a result. Yes, this carbon dioxide, it is mostly expelled. But if all carbon dioxide left our bodies, we humans would all be as thick as two planks—for part of the carbon dioxide must continually pass into our nervous system ... The nervous system needs this deadening carbon dioxide. So part of the carbon dioxide simply rises in me as interior air, and supplies my nervous system ... The breath-poison of carbon dioxide continually streams up into my head, and it is this breath-poison that enables me to think.

[118] GA 319, lecture 10, London 28.8.24
What is of a spiritual nature itself chooses carbon dioxide in order to dwell there ... On this depends the following. In the animal we have the carbon dioxide process in respiration and blood circulation—which is chiefly linked with the astral body. The astral body works—it works continually on the

carbon dioxide process. The carbon dioxide is what is outwardly, physically present in the animal, while the astral body works inwardly, spiritually. The spiritual aspect is the astral body, whose physical correlate is the carbon dioxide process underlying breathing.

[119] GA 351, lecture 3, Dornach 13.10.23

But man always produces very weak carbon dioxide, which he sends up into his head. And this prickling in the head enlivens it. It is because of this that the head is clever and not stupid. People who are really stupid . . . have too little force to link carbon with oxygen; they send no carbon upwards but link it instead with a quite different gas . . . with hydrogen . . . and then one gets methane, marsh-gas. All of us send some of this marsh-gas into our heads. We need to, otherwise we would grow too clever.

[120] GA 312, lecture 5, Dornach 25.3.20

The oyster builds up its carbonic-calcium house from within outwards. If you . . . research into the oyster from a spiritual-scientific perspective, you will come to recognize that although it is a very low form of animal life, it occupies a relatively elevated position in the whole cosmos . . . through the fact that . . . it expels what man bears within him as his thinking . . .

[121] GA 348, lecture 2, Dornach 24.10.22

The brain can also harden and calcify. It must always have a little of what occurs through the calcification process. You see, a child without a little 'chalk-sand' in his head, which the pineal gland excretes and spreads about, would stay stupid, the soul would be unable to enter, for it finds its way in through calcium. But later, when an old person has too much calcium carbonate in his system, everything hardens and he becomes senile; and then, once again, the soul is unable to get a proper grasp, for this [calcifying] is too strong . . . Then one is removed again from earthly forces.

[122] GA 319, lecture 1, Penmaenmawr 28.8.1923

Calcium carbonate remedies deriving from animal excretions . . . bring about the right relationship between the body of formative forces (ether body) and the physical body.

[123] GA 351, lecture 2, Dornach 10.10.23

Towards the feet man forms hydro-cyanic acid . . . towards the head he forms carbon dioxide . . . our head needs carbon dioxide. But this carbon dioxide meets in your head . . . with the iron in your blood . . . Once it has encountered this iron in the head, carbon dioxide then carries it everywhere into the blood . . .

[124] *Fundamentals of Therapy*, Chapter VI

See quote 115.

[125] GA 319, lecture 6, The Hague 16.11.23

See quote 116.

[126] GA 348, lecture 2, Dornach 24.10.22

See quote 121.

[127] Degenaar appendix, Hippokrates-Kalk (1922)
See quote 68.

[128] *Fundamentals of Therapy*, Chapter XVI
The organism is chiefly formed through transformation of protein substance, by means of which the latter interacts and links with mineralizing forces—as contained in calcium carbonate for example. The way the oyster forms its shell provides an image of this process. The oyster has to rid itself of what goes to make its shell, so as to retain its own protein substance. Something similar occurs in eggshell formation ... Protein process as such must be transformed into one in which are involved structuring forces that the ego organization can call forth in calcareous substance.

[129] GA 312, lecture 11, Dornach 31.3.20
In the earth process, the carbon content of the earth is a regulator for the oxygen content of the earth's environment ... The fact that the carbon content of the earth is connected with this breathing process of the earth ... In the process which occurs between the earth's carbon building process and the processes unfolding in relation to oxygen in the earth's environment lies something of what calls forth beings, entities ... etheric beings ... which continually strive away from the earth ... de-animalization of the earth ... This is why, when we introduce Carbo vegetabilis into the human organism, we are doing nothing less than administering what is striving to become animal. All symptoms ... from burping, flatulence, to putrid diarrhoea etc., from haemorrhoids on the one hand to all sorts of burning pains on the other, derive from the fact that an animal-like process—which man expelled in the course of his evolution so as to become human—is reintroduced into his organism ... if we give someone large doses of Carbo vegetabilis, we are encouraging him to defend himself against the animalization process that has entered him ...
Now the fact that we have expelled the animal from us in the course of our evolution, is connected with our possibility of actually developing ... original light. In our upper sphere we are actually original light creators, in contrast to our lower sphere where we have ... the necessary organs for defending ourselves against becoming wholly animal ...
In the human organism we really do have the possibility of wholly destroying non-human carbon in our lower sphere ... and to recreate it in its truly original form ... This renewal of carbon is connected with what we normally have within us, at the opposite pole, as light formation.
The kidneys and urinary organs participate in the breakdown of 'carbon substances'. One can enhance the whole kidney process by applying higher potencies of Carbo vegetabilis; and can then work against the course of illness that is similar to the effects of Carbo vegetabilis (in substance).

[130] GA 351, lecture 2, Dornach 10.10.23

[131] *Allgemeine und spezielle Pharmakologie und Toxikologie*, Forth, Henschler, Rummel 4.
Page 649.

[132] GA 348, lecture 2, Dornach 24.10.22
See quote 126.

[133] Gisbert Husemann, 'Das Cyan-problem und die Bewegung.' In *Erweiterung der Heilkunst*, Heft 5/59
Christoph Schulthess, 'Zur Physiologie der Bewegung und Empfindung', *Mercurstab*, Heft 3 (1989)

[134] GA 121, lecture 5, Oslo 11.6.1910
This interaction of the elements of thinking, feeling and willing [in balance—the author] initially expresses itself in such a way that this becomes the actual inner substance of love. That is what one can call the truly productive, inwardly producing aspect within earthly existence.

[135] GA 106, lecture 10, Leipzig 12.9.1908
Then human beings had to consider how they could win back the pure flow of the astral body. And there arose in the Eleusian Mysteries what was known as the search for the original purity of the astral body. One aim of the Eleusian Mysteries, and also of the Egyptians, was to recapture the astral body in its pristine golden flow. The quest of the Golden Fleece was one of the probations of the Egyptian initiations ... In the water earth [Lemuris—the author], man's astral body was permeated with golden light ...

[136] GA 93, lecture 4, Berlin 5.6.1905
When the earth was beginning to form, it was still united with the sun and what we now call the moon. The earth formed one single planetary body together with these two. First the sun separated from the earth ... and as a result ... death made its appearance ... As a consequence of the moon's departure, the division of the sexes came about in Lemurian times ... Each and everyone will reach this point at the middle of the sixth root race. But for now we are still subject to death because our etheric body has not yet attained immortality. Christianity contains the secret of how the human being can gradually evolve to the point where the etheric body resurrects [and later the physical body too—the author].

[137] Hella Wiesberger, 'Rudolf Steiner's research into the Hiram-John individuality'
See Appendix, pp. 103–06.

[138] GA 131, lecture 7, Karlsruhe 11.10.1911

[139] See Chapter 2

[140] Walter Cloos, 'Der Merkurprozess in der Natur und im Laboratorium', *Persephone 7, Heilmittel fuer typische Krankheiten nach Angaben Rudolf Steiners*, Verlag am Goetheanum 1995, pp. 377–8

[141] Walther, Cloos, 'Das Antimon in der Natur und im Laboratorium'; *Perse-*

phone 7, *Heilmittel fuer typische Krankheiten nach Angaben Rudolf Steiners*, Verlag am Goetheanum 1995, p. 175

[142] Walther Cloos, 'Von der Erdgeschichte des Eisens', *Persephone* 7, *Heilmittel fuer typische Krankheiten nach Angaben Rudolf Steiners*, Verlag am Goetheanum 1995, p. 244

[143] GA 99, lecture 7, Munich 31.5.1907

Red human blood 'could never have formed if the earth had not encountered another planet in the course of its evolution: with Mars. Before that the earth had no iron, there was no iron in the blood...'

[144] Walter Cloos, 'Von der Erdgeschichte des Eisens', *Persephone* 7, *Heilmittel fuer typische Krankheiten nach Angaben Rudolf Steiners*, Verlag am Goetheanum 1995, p. 243

[145] See Chapter 4

[146] Degenaar appendix, doctors' discussions, 6.4.24

Basically iron has, in its whole function, a similar function within the blood process to that of oxygen in the breathing process—it goes inwards ... Oxygen, with its rhythmic processes, belongs more to the breathing systems; iron belongs to the circulatory system, inasmuch as it extends into the respiratory system...

[147] Gerhard Schmidt, 'Richtlinien Rudolf Steiners zum Verstaendnis der Eisentherapie', *Persephone* 7, *Heilmittel fuer typische Krankheiten nach Angaben Rudolf Steiners*, Verlag am Goetheanum 1995, pp. 209–10

[148] See Chapter 3, Sulphur

[149] GA 312, lecture 3, Dornach 23.3.1920

Why does blood need iron? ... Because blood is the substance in the human organism that is simply ill through its very nature, and must continually be healed by iron. (Without iron the blood would continually break down and dissolve completely.)

[150] *Fundamentals of Therapy*, Chapter VII

The origins of the blood-healing effect lie in what appears as iron content when we examine red blood corpuscles ... the blood must continually endure everything of an ill-making nature; this is why it needs 'organized' iron—that is the iron, or haematin, that has been taken up into the ego organization—as continually effective remedy.

Fundamentals of Therapy, Chapter XX

Biodoron: iron for 'checking purely vital metabolic activity, which is unregulated by the ego organization'.

GA 312, lecture 20, Dornach 9.4.1920

Iron is present in the blood in order to overcome the disturbing processes which pass upwards from below; it counteracts the continual sickening of the blood through the lower organism's influence.

[151] GA 312, lecture 12, Dornach 1.4.1920

In a quite particular way Levico water unites the forces of copper, iron and arsenic: In this water, in a quite wonderful way, the dual forces of copper and iron are balanced against each other; and then, in order to once more broaden the basis of this balancing and mutual compensation, there is arsenic . . .

Represented schematically: it is as though the iron radiated positively towards the periphery, and then a negative counter-radiation came to meet it, as though hurling itself against it in spherical waves, from the force of protein.

Properly understanding the balance between iron and protein offers us an approach to all the phenomena related to anaemia in the third seven-year period. Iron mediates between what lies within our skin and what lies outside it.

GA 221, lecture 6, Dornach 11.2.1923

So in such pale, thin children, who seem to shoot upwards, we must try to lead back the hypertrophic, overactive forces in the etheric body to their proper measure, so that the human being gains weight to the body; so that, for instance, through receiving the necessary iron content, the blood gains its appropriate weight; and so that the etheric body rises upwards less, that its lifting, uprising effect is weakened.

[152] Gerhard Schmidt, 'Richtlinien Rudolf Steiners zum Verstaendnis der Eisentherapie', *Persephone 7, Heilmittel fuer typische Krankheiten nach Angaben Rudolf Steiners*, Verlag am Goetheanum 1995, pp. 217–18

[153] GA 231, lecture 3, The Hague 17.11.23

Sunspots: From the interior of the sun there is constant stimulus for sun-substance to be expelled through these dark gates into the cosmos. And what is expelled from the sun as sun-substance into the cosmos appears in the solar system as comets and meteors, also as the well-known shooting stars . . . And what is expelled into the cosmos, to the extent of assuming physical visibility as iron, becomes, in the most comprehensive way, the armour of Michael . . . If we were beings who had no iron in our blood, we would have no physical basis for unfolding the impulse to freedom . . . wherever iron appears the impulse is provided out of the cosmos, out of man, for freedom to develop . . .

GA 229, lecture 1, Dornach 5.10.1923

Shooting-star showers and iron formation in every blood corpuscle. Sulphur radiated from the nerve organization towards the brain, especially at the beginning of autumn: But into this bluish-yellow sulphur atmosphere the meteor showers stream, which are present in the life of blood. That is the other phantom. As the phantom of sulphur rises upwards like passing clouds from man's lower sphere to the head, iron formation streams straight down from the head, pouring over like meteor showers into the vital existence of the blood.

GA 348, lecture 16, Dornach 27.1.1923

... when a comet disintegrates it falls down as meteor stones, as iron ... that is also something which we have within us. When our corpses disintegrate, the iron particles of our blood are also there and are preserved. We preserve there something of our ancient comet nature. We really do what the comet does. We have iron activity in our blood because we unfold the ancient activity of cyanide.

[154] GA 351, lecture 6, Dornach 27.10.1023

The human being only begins to assimilate iron with the food he ingests ... To the extent that the infant comes to express free will, he is dependent on assimilating iron ... for this is apparent above all in those who have too little iron ... in this free will that comes to expression through language ... iron would not properly help us if we could not use it in free will ... Then the human being becomes someone who can develop his will freely and powerfully.

[155] Rudolf Hauschka, *The Nature of Substance*, Chapter 33, Rudolf Steiner Press 1983

[156] *Fundamentals of Therapy*, Chapter XVI

Gentle transition into the etheric element. Antimony preparations 'relieve protein substance of its own forces and give it the tendency to accommodate itself to the ego organization's structuring forces'.

[157] GA 312, lecture 19, Dornach 8.4.1920

Antimony forces work in blood clotting. The albuminizing (protein-building and substance-forming) forces work against antimonizing (form-creating) forces.

GA 319, lecture 1, Penmaenmawr, 28.8.1923

Enhancement of blood clotting. Antimony with its strong crystallization force works in such a way that the organism can reintegrate its astral body into the etheric body in the right way. With typhus the astral body is weak; and thus the nerve-sense organization is weakened: 'the astral body works for itself, does not properly work through into the etheric body'.

Antimony establishes the rhythm between astral and etheric bodies ...

[158] GA 319, lecture 1, Penmaenmawr, 28.8.1923

See quote 15.

[159] *Fundamentals of Therapy*, Typical remedies IV

The astral body is strengthened by the forces which continually lead to blood clotting. Typhus arises through a preponderance of the albuminizing forces...

An important remedy for use in illnesses with dangerous somnolence: In this case the formative, centrifugal forces of the astral body and thus the brain and sense processes are to some extent shut off. If one administers antimony to the organism, one artificially replaces the astral forces that are lacking ... one will always notice that antimony produces a strengthening of memory, raising of the soul's creative forces and inner

unity of soul constitution. The organism is regenerated by the strengthened soul . . .

[160] GA 319, lecture 3, London 3.9.1923

'By producing this antimony mirror, one approaches those forces which have
a reducing effect on the kinds of process that, within the metabolic system,
lead as far as the nerve processes. The antimonizing forces knock back this
process within the metabolism, which is trying to shoot beyond its goal; and
we achieve a copy or imitation of the rhythmical process through the fact
that the organic process that goes too far is driven back again by the antimony
mirror.' The 'nerve-forming process in the wrong place' (= typhus process) is
thus halted and led back to its proper place.

[161] GA 312, lecture 19, 8.4.1920

Human will forces have a destructive effect on the antimony forces, thinking
forces work together with the antimony forces ... Antimony forces are
connected with the formation of conscious, thought-force permeated will
... The 'homunculus' of ancient medicine is something like a phantom of
antimony: 'As antimony unfolded its forces, there appeared to them, pro-
jected out of their own being into the formative process they conducted
externally in their laboratories, what fights against these antimony forces as
albuminizing forces . . .'

[162] Reimar Thetter, 'Das Wesensbild des Antimon als Paradigma fuer eine
geisteswissenschaftliche HeilmittelErkenntnistheorie'; *Persephone 7, Heilmittel
fuer typische Krankheiten nach Angaben Rudolf Steiners*, Verlag am Goetheanum
1995, p. 172

[163] GA 312, lecture 19, Dornach 1.4.1920

Antimonizing force is, in planetary terms, Mercury, Venus and moon—not
working separately but together. Investigative possibilities through the fact
that 'one seeks the effect of such constellations on the human being, where
the three forces ... neutralize through the corresponding opposition and
quadrant positions ... wherever antimony (Stibium) is found on the earth,
the same force works out of the earth which works down onto the earth
from these three planetary bodies. All antimony in the earth's organization
forms a unity: the earth's overall antimony body.'

[164] Julius Metzger: *Gesichtete Homoeopathische Arzneimittellehre*, 5th edition, Haug
Verlag 1957, pp. 238–46

[165] GA 312, lecture 2, Dornach 12.4.1920

'Not too strongly diluted arsenic effects', to draw the astral body into the
physical organism, if astral body and ego were not sufficiently active within
it.

GA 313, lecture 4, Dornach 15.4.1921

Not waking up sufficiently is always a sign that the astral body is not taking
sufficient hold of the organs. Arsenic effects: these are effective if it is a matter
of treating the astral body that is already penetrated by the ego. For the astral

body alone one can consider treatments using magnetic and electrical fields.
GA 314, lecture 2, Stuttgart 1.1.1924

Arsenic basically energizes the human astral body. This is the 'archetypal effect of arsenic' and also applies to all its compounds. 'Therefore if you use arsenic, especially ... in a particular dose, you will always be able to achieve an effect if it is a question of stimulating the astral body so that it unfolds, one might say, the impulses natural to it.'

The hereditary aspect of syphilis only passes into the physical body, and is then not in the etheric body; and therefore you can, if you strongly stimulate the astral body through the use of arsenic, lead it over into the etheric body; and this would really be a quite rational way of combating it in the physical body ...
GA 317, lecture 6, Dornach 1.7.1924

Now arsenic strongly effects the flexibility of the astral body, inasmuch as the astral body strives to submerge itself, and also the form of the astral body. One can observe that the astral body of people who undertake arsenic cures slips down into the physical body.
GA 352, lecture 2, Dornach 19.1.1924

Arsenic poisoning and 'arsenic eaters': a remarkable contrast/contradiction, as one can also certainly find in nature; in one case the human being becomes thin, pale and grey-skinned, and in the other he acquires a ruddy complexion and even becomes rather plump. The human being creates arsenic within himself, just like the animal, but not the plant. Arsenic gives us the possibility of being wide awake and of sensing and feeling things; feeling arises through the fact that the astral body continually produces arsenic. Arsenic poisoning: the astral body becomes too powerful and ultimately drives life out of the organs, because a continual battle must take place in us between the astral and the etheric body. If only a little arsenic is ingested, the astral body stimulates the organs, the astral body becomes more active than previously. If the person then stops eating arsenic, the astral body grows weak and the organism quickly collapses.

[166] See quote 168.

[167] GA 313, lecture 5, Dornach, 15.4.1921

Arsenic is a remedy against excess etheric proliferation of the organs. Affinity of the astral with the etheric, and particularly through the latter to the physical body = 'arsenicization'. Gentle arsenicization, e.g. especially on awakening. We shouldn't regard 'arsenicization' in the human organism as a direct effect of arsenic itself; instead, the human being works within itself in the same way as arsenic works in the external world. Arsenicization—astralization process. When the physical organism becomes 'crumbly' and 'mummified' this is basically the same process as that of rock formation in the earth: 'there the earth is, one can say, poisoned by arsenic or at the beginning of such arsenic poisoning.'

[168] GA 312, lecture 12, Dornach 1.4.1920

On Roncegno and Levico water: 'In this water, in a quite wonderful way, the dual forces of copper and iron are balanced against each other; and then, in order to once more ... broaden the basis of this balancing and mutual compensation, arsenic is contained within in it ...

[169] GA 178, lecture 9, Dornach 25.11.17

Gold, the representative of what is sunlike within the earth's crust itself, is indeed something that conceals within itself an important secret. Gold's material relationship to other substances is actually the same as that of the idea of God to other ideas and thoughts ...

GA 157, lecture 5, Berlin 19.01.15

One could draw a comparison by saying that what gold is among metals, Michael is among the spirits in the Hierarchy of the Angeloi. All other metals work chiefly on the etheric body but gold as medicine works at the same time on the physical body ... In the same way all other leading spirits work upon the soul, but Michael can also, at the same time, work upon our physical reason and understanding.

GA 313, lecture 7, Dornach 17.4.1921

The need for a new mineral system with gold at the centre.

GA 316, lecture 8, Dornach 9.1.1924

Meditative observation of a shimmering gold disc and the independence of gold in relation to oxygen; gold and sun.

GA 97, lecture 13, Leipzig 13.10.06

There was also a time when gold was not yet solid—this was when the sun and earth were still one. When the earth departed from the sun, traces of this finer substance were still to be seen. This solidified like all metals and formed veins of gold in the rock ...

[170] GA 313, lecture 8, Dornach 18.4.1921

Gold is the balancing metal for equilibrium disorders in the heart region. It restores equilibrium to this enclosing, protective aspect and to all that is connected there with our centre. One uses Aurum in circulatory and respiratory disorders, when their cause does not lie elsewhere in the organism ...

[171] GA 312, lecture 6, Dornach 26.3.1920

'The sun maintains a condition of equilibrium between what is spiritual and what is material in the universe ... a connection between the sun and gold.' In ancient times people did not value gold for its ahrimanic value, but for its connection with the equilibrium between spirit and matter. 'The most artificial building system is already contained in gold's lustre and shining, for it is through gold that what is spiritual shines purely, as it were, into the outer world...' In ancient literature people saw in every substance the three principles of Salt, Mercury and Sulphur. 'Facilius est aurum facere quam destruere.'

[172] GA 202, lecture 12, Dornach 19.12.1920

Just as we attain freedom when the life of thinking is penetrated and permeated with will, so we come to love when the life of will is imbued with thoughts. In our actions we develop love by allowing our thoughts to pour into the life of will; we develop freedom in our thinking by allowing the will element to radiate into our thoughts. And since we are a whole, a totality, as human beings, when we manage to find freedom in our life of thinking and love in our life of will, so freedom will participate in our actions, and love in our thinking. They permeate one another and we accomplish deeds, thought-filled deeds in love, and a will-imbued thinking from which actions, in turn, arise in freedom.

'So you see how the two highest ideals of freedom and love grow together within the human being.'

[173] GA 312, lecture 3, Dornach 23.3.1920

See quote 149.

[174] GA 312, lecture 10, Dornach 30.3.1920

Indication that the formative forces of gold create a balance between man's more central realm (Cu, Hg, Ag) and his more peripheral realm (Pb, Sn, Fe).

[175] GA 265, lecture, Munich 21.5.1907

See this book, Appendix: Rudolf Steiner on Carbo and the Philosopher's Stone

[176] GA 265, lecture, Munich, 21.5.1907

See this book, Appendix: Rudolf Steiner on Carbo and the Philosopher's Stone

[177] GA 232, lecture 14, Dornach 23.12.23

When the pupil sinks his soul-imbued gaze into direct but diminished sunlight, this prepares him for understanding the gold of the earth ... It has no direct relation to the etheric or astral body, but a direct relation to what lies in human thinking ... And when gold is administered in the right dose to the human organism it restores strength of thinking. It restores to thinking a power which enables it to work down into the astral body and even into the etheric. Gold enlivens us through thinking ... By means of gold the ego organization becomes able to work down into the etheric body ... The etheric body can in turn work upon the physical body. But gold actually allows us to powerfully sustain our thoughts right down into the etheric body.

[178] GA 93, lecture 2, Berlin 22.5.1905

Between the second and the sixth root race the earth separated off; in the third the moon separated. Now the earth is evolving from the third to the sixth root race, when the sun will once more be united with the earth. Then a new epoch will begin, once man has arrived at a much higher level and no longer incarnates ... The sun uniting with the earth is heralded by the appearance of Christ on earth ...

[179] GA 93, lecture 18, Berlin 2.1.1906

By nature the man represents the force which creates in the non-living realm, while the woman is representative of the living, creative forces through which the human race continues to evolve from its natural basis. This contrast must be overcome ...

[180] A description of how the two pillars are connected with birth and death is to be found in the lecture given in Kassel on 7 July 1909. Also the paintings in the large cupola of the first Goetheanum (in the threefold motive 'I–A–O' over the archway above the stage) points to this connection of the portfolio of twelve sketches for the paintings of the large cupola of the first Goetheanum and the book by Hilde Raske, *Das Farbenwort*.

[181] In the lecture given in Dornach 29 December 1918, it is pointed out that the pillars in the present-day occult societies can no longer be erected in the proper fashion, and should also not be erected, because the proper setting can only be found when a true, inwardly experienced initiation takes place. In addition to that one is not able to erect them as they should be erected in the case where a person through death or initiation leaves his body.

[182] See the lecture in Berlin, 14 December 1911 and *The Gospel of St Mark* (GA 139)

BIBLIOGRAPHY

Rudolf Steiner, *Knowledge of the Higher Worlds—How is it Achieved?* Rudolf Steiner Press 1993. Also available as: *How to Know Higher Worlds*, Anthroposophic Press 1994

Rudolf Steiner, *Occult Science: An Outline*, Rudolf Steiner Press, London, 1963. Chapter IV, 'Man and the evolution of world'. Also available as: *An Outline of Esoteric Science*, Anthroposophic Press 1997

Rudolf Steiner and Ita Wegman, *Fundamentals of Therapy*, Chapters VI, VII, XIII, XIV, XV, XVI, XVII, XIX, XX. Typical remedies IV. Current edition: *Extending Practical Medicine*, Rudolf Steiner Press 1996

Degenaar, Phosphor und Kalzium (1922), Hippocrates-Kalk (1922). Appendix, doctors' discussions, 6.4.24. (A collection of case studies of patients treated with support and advice from Rudolf Steiner. Private printing.)

Persephone 7, Heilmittel fuer typische Krankheiten nach Angaben Rudolf Steiners, Verlag am Goetheanum 1995:

Walter Cloos, 'Der Merkurprozess in der Natur und im Laboratorium'

Walther Cloos, 'Das Antimon in der Natur und im Laboratorium'

Walther Cloos, 'Von der Erdgeschichte des Eisens'

Gerhard Schmidt, 'Richtlinien Rudolf Steiners zum Verstaendnis der Eisentherapie'

Reimar Thetter, 'Das Wesensbild des Antimon als Paradigma fuer eine geisteswissenschaftliche Heilmittel-Erkenntnistheorie'

Rudolf Hauschka, *The Nature of Substance*, Chapter 33, Rudolf Steiner Press 1983

Ala Selawry, *Metallfuktionstypen in Psychologie und Medizin*, Haug Verlag, Stuttgart. Zinn-Kapitel

Ala Selawry, *Metallfuktionstypen in Psychologie und Medizin*. Haug Verlag, Stuttgart. Blei-, Zinn- und Eisen-Kapitel

Beiträge zur Rudolf Steiner Gesamtausgabe, Heft 20, Seite 20

Beiträge zur Rudolf Steiner Gesamtausgabe, Heft 35, Seite 13

Allgemeine und spezielle Pharmakologie und Toxikologie, Forth, Henschler, Rummel, 4. Auflage

Gisbert Husemann, 'Das Cyan-problem und die Bewegung', in *Beiträge zur Erweiterung der Heilkunst*, Heft 5/59

Christoph Schulthess, 'Zur Physiologie der Bewegung und Empfindung', in *Mercurstab*, Heft 3 (1989)

Julius Metzger: *Gesichtete Homoeopathische Arzneimittellehre*, 5th edition, Haug Verlag 1957, pp. 238–46

Lectures by Rudolf Steiner

RSP = Rudolf Steiner Press
AP = Anthroposophic Press

GA 58, Munich 14.3.1909: in *Metamorphosis of the Soul*, Volume 2 (RSP 1983)

GA 93, Berlin 16.12.1904, 22.5.1905, 29.5.1905, 5.6.1905, 21.10.1905, 2.1.1906: in *The Temple Legend* (RSP 1997)

GA 93a, Berlin 29.9.1905, 3.11.1905: in *Foundation of Esotericism* (RSP 1983)

GA 95, Stuttgart 31.8.1906: in *Founding a Science of the Spirit* (RSP 1999)

GA 97, Leipzig 13.10.06, 16.2.1907: not translated

GA 99, Munich 25.5.1907, 29.5.1907, 31.5.1907, 6.6.1907: in *Rosicrucian Wisdom* (RSP 1999)

GA 100, Kassel 9.6.07: not translated

GA 104, Nuremberg 18.6.1908: in *Apocalypse of St John* (RSP 1985)

GA 106, Leipzig 7.9.1908, 8.9.1908, 12.9.1908: in *Egyptian Myths and Mysteries* (AP 1971)

GA 107, Berlin 19.10.1908, 21.10.1908: not translated

GA 112, Kassel 30.6.1909 in: *The Gospel of St John in Relation to the other Gospels* (AP 1982)

GA 121, Oslo 11.6.1910 in: *The Mission of the Individual Folk Souls* (RSP 1970)

GA 128, Prague 22.3.1911, 26.3.1911, 27.3.1911: in *An Occult Physiology* (RSP 1983)

GA 131, Karlsruhe 10.10.1911, 13.10.1911: in *From Jesus to Christ* (RSP 1991)

GA 132, Berlin 7.11.1911: in *Spiritual Hierarchies and the Physical World* (AP 1996)

GA 136, Helsinki 11.4.1912, 13.4.1912: in *Spiritual Beings in the Heavenly Bodies* (AP 1992)

GA 145, The Hague 29.3.1913: in *Effects of Esoteric Development* (AP 1997)

GA 157, Berlin, 19.01.15: in *The Destinies of Individuals and Nations* (RSP 1986)

GA 178, Dornach 25.11.17: in *Wrong and Right Use of Esoteric Knowledge* (RSP 1966)

GA 202, Dornach 19.12.1920: in *The Bridge Between Universal Spirituality and the Physical Constitution of Man* (AP 1979)

GA 208, Dornach 30.10.21: in *Cosmosophy*, Vol. 2 (Completion Press, Australia, 1997)

GA 213, Dornach 2.7.22: in *Human Questions and Cosmic Answers* (Anthroposophical Publishing Co. 1960)

GA 218, Dornach 20.10.22: not translated

GA 221, Dornach 11.2.1923: in *Earthly Knowledge and Heavenly Wisdom* (AP 1991)

GA 227, Penmaenmawr 29.8.23: in *The Evolution of Consciousness* (RSP 1991)

GA 229, Dornach 5.10.1923: not translated

GA 230, Dornach 9.11.1923, 10.11.1923, 11.11.1923: in *Harmony of the Creative Word* (RSP 2001)

GA 231, The Hague, 17.11.23: in *At Home in the Universe* (AP 2000)

GA 232, Dornach 23.12.23: in *Mystery Knowledge and Mystery Centres* (RSP 1997)

GA 233, Dornach 30.12.23: in *World History and the Mysteries in the Light of Anthroposophy* (RSP 1997)

GA 235, Dornach 1.3.24: in *Karmic Relationships*, Vol 1 (RSP 1972)

GA 239, Breslau 14.6.24: in *Karmic Relationships*, Vol 7 (RSP 1973)

GA 245, Berlin 2.10.1906: not translated

GA 265, Munich 21.5.1907: not translated

GA 284, Munich 19.5.1907: not translated

GA 312, Dornach 23.3.1920, 25.3.1920, 26.3.1920, 30.3.1920, 31.3.20, 1.4.1920, 9.4.1920: in *Introducing Anthroposophical Medicine* (AP 1999)

GA 313, Dornach 15.4.1921, 17.4.1921, 18.4.1921: in *Anthroposophical Spiritual Science and Medical Therapy* (Mercury Press 1991)

GA 314, Dornach 7.4.1920, 9.10.1920: in *Physiology and Therapeutics* (Mercury Press 1986). Stuttgart 1.1.1924: not translated

GA 316, Dornach 4.1.1924, 9.1.1924: in *Course for Young Doctors* (Mercury Press, New York 1994)

GA 317, Dornach 25.6.24, 30.6.1924, 1.7.1924, 2.7.1924, 3.7.1924: in *Education for Special Needs* (RSP 1998)

GA 318, Dornach 11.9.1924, 13.9.1924, 14.9.1924, 18.9.1924: in *Pastoral Medicine* (AP 1987)

GA 319, Penmaenmawr 28.8.1923, London 3.9.1923, The Hague 16.11.1923, Arnheim 24.7.24, London 29.8.24 in: *The Healing Process* (AP 2000)

GA 327, Koberwitz 7.6.1924, 10.6.1924, 11.6.1924: in *Agriculture* (Bio-dynamic Farming and Gardening Association, Kimberton)

GA 347, Dornach 9.8.1922, 16.9.1922: in *The Human Being in Body, Soul and Spirit* (AP/RSP 1989)

GA 348, Dornach 24.10.1922, 27.1.1923: in *From Comets to Cocaine ...* (RSP 2000)

GA 349, Dornach 21.2.1923 in: *From Limestone to Lucifer ...* (RSP 1999)

GA 351, Dornach 10.10.1923, 13.10.23: not translated. Dornach 27.10.1923 in: *Cosmic Workings in Earth and Man* (Rudolf Steiner Publishing Co. 1952). Dornach 1.12.23, 5.12.23: in *Bees* (AP 1998)

GA 352, Dornach 19.1.1924: in *From Elephants to Einstein ...* (RSP 1988)

GA 354, Dornach 3.7.1924: in *Evolution of the Earth and Man* (AP/RSP 1987)